Step by Step®
INTERVENTIONAL ULTRASOUND IN OBSTETRICS AND GYNECOLOGY

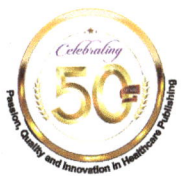

Step by Step®
INTERVENTIONAL ULTRASOUND IN OBSTETRICS AND GYNECOLOGY

Second Edition

Editor-in-Chief

Narendra Malhotra
MD FICMCH FICOG FRCOG FICS FMAS FIAP
President, INSARG, Past President, FOGSI/IFUMB/ISPAT/ISAR
Vice President, WAPM/SAFOG
Managing Director, Global Rainbow Health Care & MNMH(P) Ltd
Agra, Uttar Pradesh, India
Professor, Sarajevo School of Science and Technology, Croatia

Associate Editors

Nidhi Gupta MS FICMCH FICOG
Past President, Agra Obstetrical & Gynecological Society
Professor, Department of Obstetrics and Gynecology
SN Medical College, Agra, Uttar Pradesh, India

Neharika Malhotra
MD (Gold Medalist) DRM (Germany) FICMCH
Fellow ICOG (Rep Med) ICOG (USG)
Joint Secretary, FOGSI, Chair YTP Committee, FOGSI
Director and Consultant, Global Rainbow IVF & MNMH(P) Ltd
Agra, Uttar Pradesh, India

Jaideep Malhotra
MD FICMCH FICOG FRCOG FRCPI FMAS
President, SAFOM/ISPAT
Past President, IMS/ISAR/FOGSI/ASPIRE
Managing Director, ART—Global Rainbow IVF & MNMH(P) Ltd
Agra, Uttar Pradesh, India

Kuldeep Singh MBBS FAUI FICMCH
Consultant Ultrasonologist
Dr Kuldeep's Ultrasound and Color Doppler Clinic
New Delhi, India

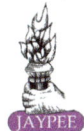

JAYPEE BROTHERS MEDICAL PUBLISHERS
The Health Sciences Publisher
New Delhi | London

Jaypee Brothers Medical Publishers (P) Ltd

Headquarters
Jaypee Brothers Medical Publishers (P) Ltd
EMCA House, 23/23-B
Ansari Road, Daryaganj
New Delhi 110 002, India
Landline: +91-11-23272143, +91-11-23272703
+91-11-23282021, +91-11-23245672
Email: jaypee@jaypeebrothers.com

Corporate Office
Jaypee Brothers Medical Publishers (P) Ltd
4838/24, Ansari Road, Daryaganj
New Delhi 110 002, India
Phone: +91-11-43574357
Fax: +91-11-43574314
Email: jaypee@jaypeebrothers.com

Overseas Office
J.P. Medical Ltd
83 Victoria Street, London
SW1H 0HW (UK)
Phone: +44 20 3170 8910
Fax: +44 (0)20 3008 6180
Email: info@jpmedpub.com

Website: www.jaypeebrothers.com
Website: www.jaypeedigital.com

© 2021, Jaypee Brothers Medical Publishers

The views and opinions expressed in this book are solely those of the original contributor(s)/author(s) and do not necessarily represent those of editor(s) of the book.

All rights reserved. No part of this publication may be reproduced, stored or transmitted in any form or by any means, electronic, mechanical, photocopying, recording or otherwise, without the prior permission in writing of the publishers.

All brand names and product names used in this book are trade names, service marks, trademarks or registered trademarks of their respective owners. The publisher is not associated with any product or vendor mentioned in this book.

Medical knowledge and practice change constantly. This book is designed to provide accurate, authoritative information about the subject matter in question. However, readers are advised to check the most current information available on procedures included and check information from the manufacturer of each product to be administered, to verify the recommended dose, formula, method and duration of administration, adverse effects and contraindications. It is the responsibility of the practitioner to take all appropriate safety precautions. Neither the publisher nor the author(s)/editor(s) assume any liability for any injury and/or damage to persons or property arising from or related to use of material in this book.

This book is sold on the understanding that the publisher is not engaged in providing professional medical services. If such advice or services are required, the services of a competent medical professional should be sought.

Every effort has been made where necessary to contact holders of copyright to obtain permission to reproduce copyright material. If any have been inadvertently overlooked, the publisher will be pleased to make the necessary arrangements at the first opportunity. The **CD/DVD-ROM** (if any) provided in the sealed envelope with this book is complimentary and free of cost. **Not meant for sale.**

Inquiries for bulk sales may be solicited at: jaypee@jaypeebrothers.com

Step by Step® Interventional Ultrasound in Obstetrics and Gynecology

First Edition: 2004

Second Edition: **2021**

ISBN: 978-93-5270-903-8

__Dedicated to__
All the ultrasound lovers

Preface to the Second Edition

*"Use sound to see better
Turn on the color to improve your image
Shift to the 3rd and 4th dimension
Heal with sound"*

Ultrasound today is the mainstay in the field of obstetrics and gynecology.

Introduction of interventional procedures in obstetrics and gynecology has now made it possible to make histopathological diagnosis.

After the huge success of the first edition of this book we have come out with the second edition with addition of commonly used interventional procedures.

The procedures have been simplified step by step for the practitioners to learn and practice in their patients.

Narendra Malhotra
Nidhi Gupta
Neharika Malhotra
Jaideep Malhotra
Kuldeep Singh

Preface to the First Edition

Ultrasound today is the mainstay investigation in the field of obstetrics and gynecology. It is now quick, easy, reproducible and inexpensive to make an anatomical diagnosis in obstetrics and gynecology. The addition of color gives us an insight to the physiology of the area/organ/fetus being scanned and 3D and 4D have added a new anatomical plane and dimension.

Introduction of interventional procedures to obstetrics and gynecological ultrasound has now made it possible for us to help in making a histopathological diagnosis.

This step by step book aims at introducing the reader and familiarizing the reader to interventional sonography in Obstetrics and Gynecology.

It is mandatory by the Indian PNDT law to register your machine and clinic to perform interventional genetic diagnostic procedures.

Kuldeep Singh
Narendra Malhotra

Acknowledgments

Our heartiest thanks to our parents, elders, teachers, spouses, siblings, our sons, daughters and our friends who have helped us step by step at every step of our ambitious project of step by step series.

We were introduced to interventional sonography by Ananda Kumar (Singapore), Rajat Goswamy (UK), Asim Kurjak and Sanja Kupesic (Croatia), Prof Alfred Kratrochwil (Austria), Ashok Khurana, Ambarish Dalal, Pratap Kumar, Bhupendra Ahuja, Dr PK Shah, Jatin P Shah and Pranay Shah and many others who taught us small tricks of the trade at each step of our life.

We are indebted to Prof Struat Campbell and Prof Asim Kurjak for teaching us imaging and grateful to Ian Donald School, India and INSUOG.

Special thanks to Dr Rahul Gupta and Nitin Agarwal of Rainbow 4D imaging center for all the images.

Editor-in-Chief
Narendra Malhotra

Contents

1. Introduction 1
2. Training 9
3. Patient Counseling, Ethical and Legal Issues 16
4. Interventional Ultrasound in Daily Obstetrical-Gynecological Practice 26
5. Obstetric Procedures—Overview 30
6. Anesthesia for Interventional Ultrasound in Obstetrics.... 53
7. Ultrasound-guided Techniques in Fetal Medicine 59
8. Coelocentesis 65
9. Chorionic Villus Sampling... 69
10. Amniocentesis 77
11. Multifetal Reduction... 84
12. Prenatal Diagnosis and Therapeutic Techniques in Twin Pregnancies 93
13. Gynecology Procedures 98
14. Ultrasound in Treatment of Adnexal Cystic Masses 115
15. Transvaginal Sonographic Puncture Procedures for Management of Ectopic Pregnancies 121
16. Ultrasound-guided Transcervical Metroplasty................ 130
17. Infertility Procedures.. 138
18. Techniques for Assisted Reproduction 155

APPENDICES

Appendix 1: Ectopic Pregnancy Pretreatment Scores 163

Appendix 2: High Risk Pregnancy Evaluation Form 165

Appendix 3: Consent Form for IVF-ET 172

Index *191*

CHAPTER 1

Introduction

FILLING FORMS

Maintain a form for further follow-up in your clinic. One never knows when the information is required.

The routine information required in these forms is:
a. Name
b. Age
c. Address
d. Telephone Number
e. Referred by
f. PNDT Act Form 'F' as required by Government of India law
g. Undertaking by patient and doctor for obstetric ultrasound with Form 'F' and Form 'G'
h. For genetic defects for interventional procedures, the clinic has to be specially registered and licensed by Government under the PNDT Act as a genetic Lab.

RELEVANT HISTORY

Always spend few minutes with your patient to take the details of the history. It gives confidence to the patient and you get your perspective of what all to expect.

The history to be taken routinely is:
- Previous obstetric history consisting of details of any abortions (spontaneous or missed), any second or third

trimester losses (possible reasons), any previous deliveries (vaginal or caesarian). Try and look into the previous records which can throw any light
- Any symptoms in this pregnancy
- Any ultrasound done so far in this pregnancy. Check the records carefully
- Last menstrual period and regularity of menstrual cycles.
- Any tests done and their reports
- Referring doctors requisition slip (This is now a legal requirement with Form 'F').

MACHINE AND EQUIPMENT (FIGS 1.1 TO 1.5)

Any good resolution scanner is a requisite for interventional procedures and should have all the probes (transabdominal and transvaginal) all standard accessories, biopsy guides for both probes, recording and documenting facility and different types of needles, etc.

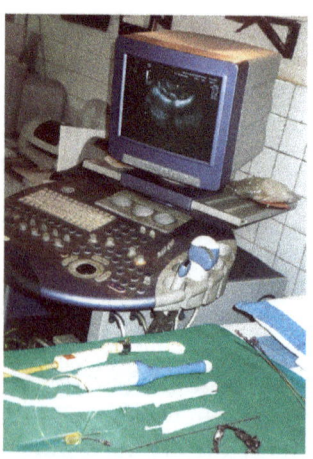

Fig. 1.1: Machine with probes and biopsy guide.

Introduction

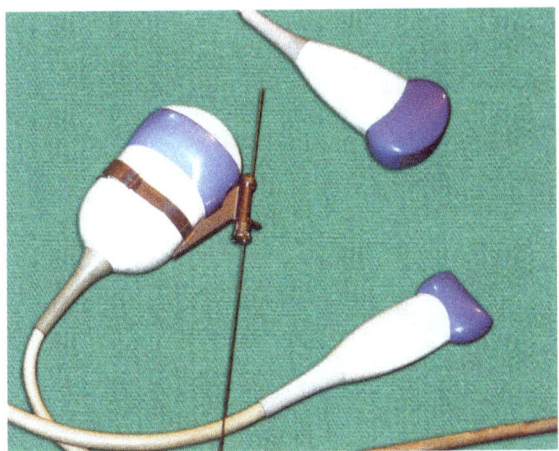

Fig. 1.2: Abdominal probes with biopsy guide and needle.

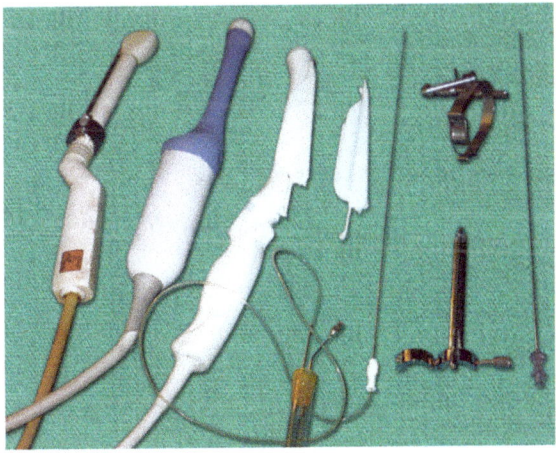

Fig. 1.3: Vaginal probes and biopsy guides with needles.

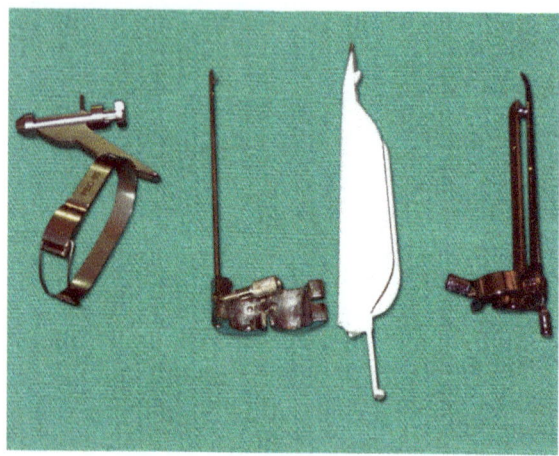

Fig. 1.4: Various biopsy guides.

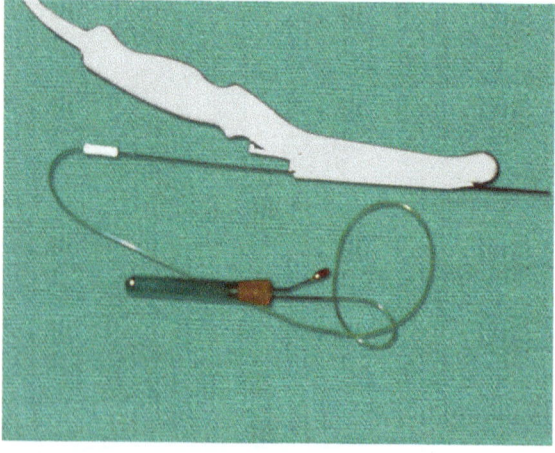

Fig. 1.5: Ovum pick up set.

- Machine with transabdominal and transvaginal probes
- Minor operation theatre
- Biopsy guides for transabdominal and transvaginal probes.
- Biopsy needles of all sizes and lumen for abdominal and vaginal routes
- Standard accessories
- Standard equipment for minor OT procedure
- Consent form.

PATIENT PREPARATIONS

Patient is prepared for as any other minor operative procedures.
- Admission charts and proper consent
- Preoperative antibiotic and Tetvac injection
- Preoperative part preparation, bowel and bladder evacuation
- Supine/lithotomy position
- Sterilized probe (Dipping in Cidex solution)
- Aseptic measures
- Analgesia/anesthesia.

COUNSELING AND LEGAL ASPECTS

- Proper genetic registered center (PNDT Act)
- Genetic screening (Flowchart 1.1A)
- Genetic counseling for chromosomal defects
- Counseling for procedure and side effects (Flowchart 1.1B).
- Legal consent
- Counseling for acceptable procedure-related risks and abortions (Pre and post-test counceling)
- Legal malpractices issues may be different in different countries (MTP laws).

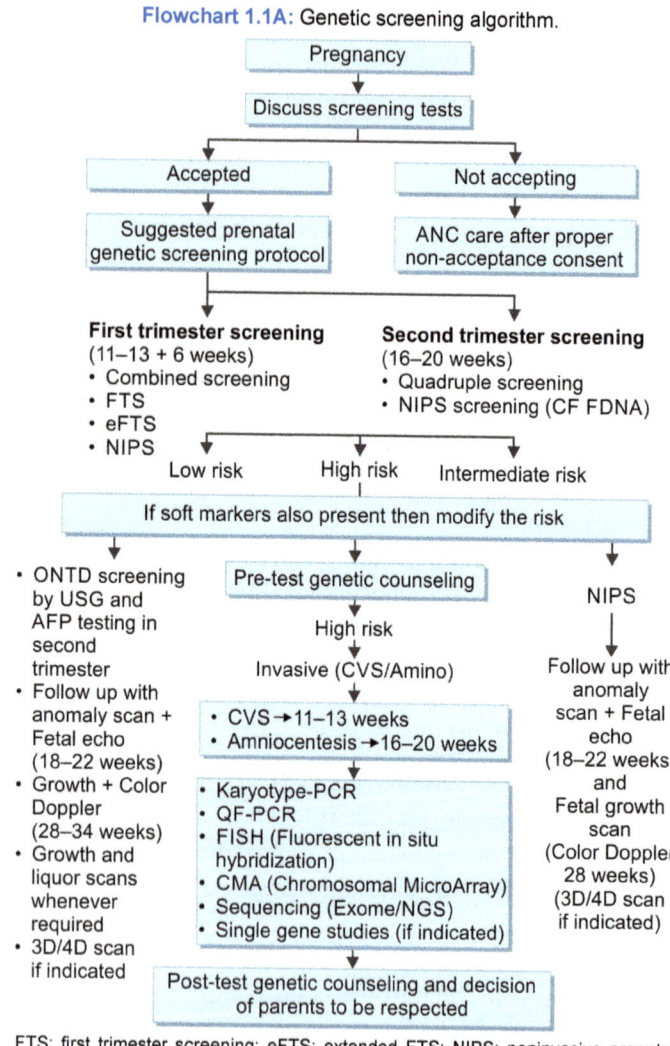

Flowchart 1.1A: Genetic screening algorithm.

FTS: first trimester screening; eFTS: extended FTS; NIPS: noninvasive prenatal screening; CF-DNA: cell free DNA; ONTD: open neural tube defects; USG: ultrasonography; AFP: alpha-fetoprotein; CVS: chorion villus sampling.

Flowchart 1.1B: Approach to a pregnant patient for anomaly detection and confirmation.

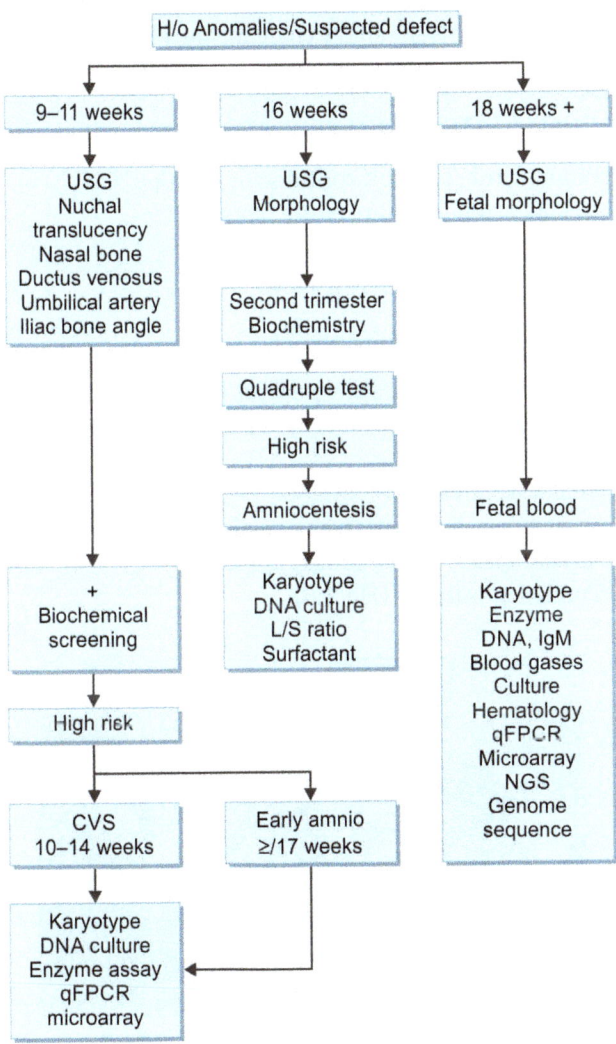

Note: A plaintiff must demonstrate that the physician breached the standard care and his action/inaction caused injury, since the standard care is so rapidly changing the physician must be alert to new developments and must inform these to the patient.

DOCUMENTATION AND REPORTING

- Proper hard copy/soft copy documentation
- Detailed step-wise procedure reporting
- Report complications
- Clear follow-up of instructions.

ANALGESIA AND ANESTHESIA

Usually these procedures are quick and relatively painless and require only reassurance, mild analgesia and local anesthesia.
- Local anesthesia
- Analgesic injections
- Short general anesthesia with propofol, pentothal or ketamine
- All standard resuscitation equipment
- Trained anesthetist (Fig. 1.6).

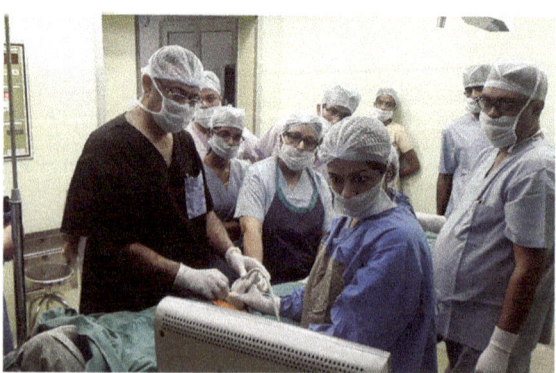

Fig. 1.6: Amniocentesis and training of students

CHAPTER 2

Training

A proper training in obstetric and gynecological ultrasound is a must and a postgraduate degree/diploma in obstetric and gynecology/surgery/Interventional Radiology/Radiology/MBBS with one year training under a Radiologist (see PCPNT Law India). Must have performed 20 procedures under guidance.

GUIDELINES

The practice of ultrasound and the use of diagnostic and interventional ultrasound is now a necessary tool rather than a luxury. It is impossible to even conceive an Obstetric Care Unit and Fetal Medicine Unit or even Gynecology and Infertility Diagnostic Unit without ultrasound.

To practice ultrasound in India it is mandatory to be trained in ultrasonography under proper guides (PCPNT Law).

THEORETICAL ASPECTS

The theoretical aspects one should know, should cover topics on Physics of ultrasound, ultrasound machines and probes, how to use an ultrasound machine, PNDT Act, laws of ultrasound, medicolegal aspects, methodology, patient preparations, complete obstetric ultrasound uses including use in first, second and third trimesters, diagnosis of threatened abortion, ectopic pregnancy, biometry, anomaly scanning, IUGR, placental evaluation, amniotic fluid evaluation, color Doppler uses and 3D and 4D ultrasound.

Complete gynecological ultrasound aspects include use of TVS, color Doppler and 3D in evaluating female pelvis and evaluating infertility and complete interventional procedures.

TRAINING PARAMETERS (PROPOSED)

First Level

(At least 30 hours a week for two months)
These are aimed at to:
- Confirm intrauterine pregnancy
- Confirm viability
- Determine number of gestations
- Fetal biometry
- Assessment of growth
- Presentation
- Amniotic fluid assessment
- Placental assessment
- Cervix measurement
- Suspect abnormalities.

Second Level

(About 100 sessions and 300 hours)
These are aimed at to:
- Detect and specify early pregnancy problems
- Detect and specify abnormalities
- Assessment of growth restriction
- Fetal biophysical profiling
- Understanding Color Doppler
- Accurately sampling various blood vessels by Doppler and analyzing them

- Knowledge of interventional procedure
- Knowledge of 3D and 4D
- Analysis of malignancies.

Third Level (3 years)

These are aimed at to:
- Acquire 3D and 4D image
- Perform interventional procedures
- Research and development
- Acquire ability to teach basic skills.

SUGGESTED TRAINING SCHEDULE

Viable pregnancies	10
Nonviable pregnancies	10
Normal biometry	10
Growth restrictions	10
Abnormal pregnancy (Ectopic/Multiple etc.)	10
Color Doppler Studies Obstetric	10
Color Doppler Studies Gynae	10
IUCD's	5
Fibroids	10
Ovarian cysts	10
Gynae disorders	10
Transvaginal scan	10

These are minimum number of scans for Level-I training.

Another 100 cases of detailed Obstetric and Gynecological cases for various indications including color and 3-D should be logged for Level-II training.

A standard reporting format for Gynecology and Obstetrics should be adhered to with details of different descriptive terminology.

PREREQUISITE CRITERIA FOR A TRAINED ULTRASONOLOGIST

- The ultrasonologist should be able to identify early pregnancy and emergency gynecological problems by transvaginal and transabdominal ultrasound.
  - Early pregnancy:
    - Fetal viability
    - Description of the gestational sac, embryo, yolk sac
    - Single and multiple gestation (chorionicity).
  - Pathology:
    - Early pregnancy failure
    - Ectopic pregnancy
    - Gross fetal abnormalities such as nuchal translucency, hydropic abnormalities
    - Hydatidiform mole
    - Associated pelvic tumors
    - First trimester markers of chromosomal anomalies.
  - Gynecology:
    - Normal pelvic anatomy
    - Uterine size and endometrial thickness
    - Measurement of ovaries
    - Pelvic tumors, e.g., fibroids, cysts hydrosalpinx
    - Peritoneal fluid
    - Intrauterine contraceptive devices.
- The ultrasonologist should be able to recognize the following normal fetal anatomical features from 18 weeks onwards by abdominal ultrasound.
  - Shape of the skull: Nuchal skinfold
  - Brain: Ventricles, cerebellum, choroid plexus
  - Facial profile
  - Spine: Both longitudinally and transversely

- Heart rate and rhythm, size and position, four-chamber view
- Size and morphology of the lungs
- Shape of the thorax and abdomen
- Abdomen: Diaphragm, stomach, liver and umbilical vein, kidneys, abdominal wall and umbilicus
- Limbs: Femur, tibia and fibula, humerus, radius and ulna, feet and hands—these to include shape, echogenicity and movement
- Multiple pregnancy: Monochorionic and dichorionic, twin-twin transfusion syndrome
- Amount of amniotic fluid
- Placental location
- Cord and number of vessels.
* Fetal biometry
    - Crown-rump length, biparietal diameter, femur length, head circumference, abdominal circumference, interpretation of growth charts.
* Activity: Recognize and quantify
    - Fetal movements
    - Breathing movements
    - Eye movements.
* Second trimester markers of chromosomal anomalies and their scoring.

MANDATORY PROPOSED CERTIFICATION FOR AN ULTRASONOLOGIST (OBS AND GYN) (SEE PCPNT LAW)

1. One hundred hours in 6 months, of supervised scanning to include (one year observership):
    a. 100 gynecological examinations and early pregnancy problems (principally by transvaginal sonography but transabdominal experience also required)

b. 200 obstetric scans covering the full spectrum of obstetric conditions.
2. Logbooks:

 30 cases on one A4 page with ultrasound picture, at least 15 anomalies should be included.

These are suggested training hours and comply with the Indian Government's requirement under the modified PNDT Act.

GYNECOLOGICAL ULTRASOUND

- Normal pelvic anatomy
  - Uterus
    - Uterine size, position, shape and movement
    - Cyclical morphological changes in the endometrium
    - Measurement of endometrial thickness.
  - Ovaries
    - Size, position, shape and measurement
    - Cyclical morphological changes
    - Measurement of follicles and corpus luteum
    - Assessment of peritoneal fluid.
- Gynecological complications:
  - Uterus
    - Fibroids
    - Adenomyosis
    - Endometrial hyperplasia
    - Endometrial cancer
    - Polyps
    - Location of intrauterine contraceptive device.
  - Tubes
    - Hydrosalpinx and other abnormalities of the fallopian tubes

- Ovaries
  - Cysts; benign and malignant, morphological scoring systems
  - Endometriosis
  - Ovarian carcinoma
  - Differential diagnosis of pelvic masses.
- Infertility:
  - Monitoring of follicular development in spontaneous and stimulated cycles
    - Diagnosis of hyperstimulation syndrome
    - Diagnosis of polycystic ovaries
    - Sonosalpingography.
- Invasive procedures:
  - Oocyte retrieval
  - Injection of ovarian cysts
  - Aspiration of ovarian cysts
  - Drainage of pelvic abscesses
  - Extraction of intrauterine contraceptive device.
- Doppler in gynecology
- Infertility and oncology.

TRAINING

Training certification as accepted by PNDT law should be taken before attempting any interventional procedure. Proper training and experience can be gained by regular practice on Phantoms. Operator must be well familiar with all probes and needles.

The center should be registered in PCPNDT and all necessary equipment should be in the center. It is advisable to work with good resolution machines.

3
CHAPTER

Patient Counseling, Ethical and Legal Issues

GENETIC COUNSELING

Many interventional obstetrical procedures are performed to identify increased risks for birth and genetic disorders prenatally.

The American Society of Human Genetic has used a statement defining the appropriate goals and content of genetic counseling.

Pre-procedure genetic counseling is a communication process which deals with the human problems associated with the occurrence or the risk of occurrence, of a genetic disorder in a family. This process involves an attempt by one or more trained persons to help the individual or family to:
- Comprehend the medical facts, including the diagnosis, probable course of the disorder and the available management
- Appreciates the way heredity contributes to the disorder, and the risk of recurrence in specified relatives
- Understand the alternatives for dealing with the risk of recurrence
- Choose the course of action which seems to their appropriate in view of their risk, their family goals, and their ethical and religious standards, and to act in accordance with the decision. To make the best possible adjustment

to the disorder in an affected family member and/or to the risk of recurrence of that disorder.

All pregnancies should be offered antenatal screening (Figs. 3.1A and B)

COUNSELING PATIENTS PRIOR TO INTERVENTIONAL ULTRASOUND (PRE AND POST TEXT COUNCELING)

It is important, that, a very appropriate indication is available to the physician before offering an interventional procedure with any degree of risk to the mother, fetus or the patient.

Until a substantial data is available and risk benefit of an interventional procedure is documented; the procedure should be restricted and not universally applied.

The patient before undergoing the interventional procedure should be made aware of the short and long term risks of the procedure and the extent of the data of which this risk assessment is made and the limitations of the data.

The patients also be informed of the realistic appraisal of possible and likely benefits, accuracy of diagnostic tests to be utilized and a discussion of alternatives.

This counseling should preferably be done in a close chamber, giving it appropriate time, one to one discussion (face to face) with eye contact.

The counselor should be well aware of the facts and should be prepared with the data and to answer judiciously any query done by the patients (Fig. 3.1A).

COUNSELING IN FETAL MEDICINE

Invasive procedures performed during pregnancy differ from procedures in any other medical setting, as there are two patients potentially at risk—the mother and the fetus.

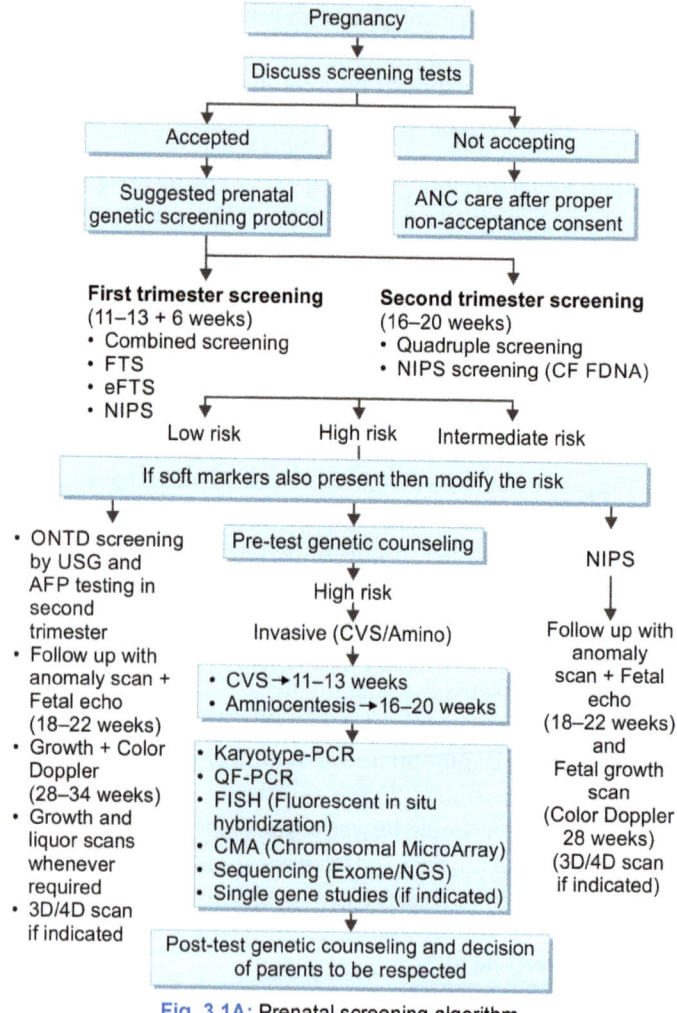

Fig. 3.1A: Prenatal screening algorithm.
FTS: first trimester screening; eFTS: extended FTS; NIPS: noninvasive prenatal screening; CF-DNA: cell free DNA; ONTD: open neural tube defects; USG: ultrasonography; AFP: alpha-fetoprotein; CVS: chorion villus sampling.

Patient Counseling, Ethical and Legal Issues

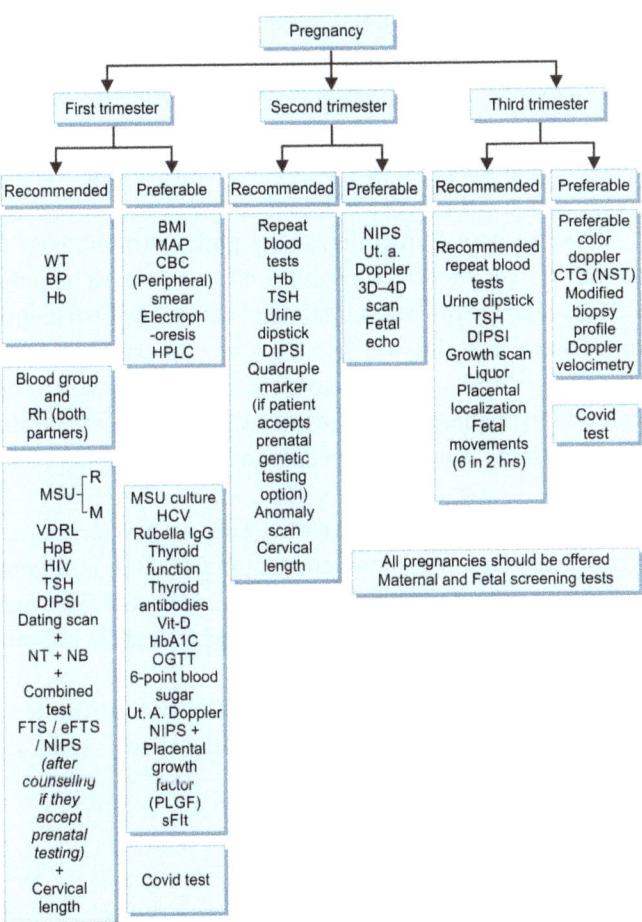

Fig. 3.1B: Prenatal screening algorithm.

Although, the physician's primary obligation is to the mother but all efforts should be directed to safeguard the health of the fetus.

The counselor must be non-directional and must inform the patient of the possible risks of the procedure, alternative procedures and the risks and benefits of all.

It would be worthwhile for the patient to choose the procedure over another, though the counselor must help the patient to decide the safest method of achieving the patient's reproductive goal. The decision regarding the procedure also depends on the relative risk/benefit of a high risk patient for an abnormality; patient's past pregnancy experience or and the perceived importance of procedure induced fetal loss or fetal defects.

Counseling patients who have been offered new techniques for fetal therapy like open/endoscopic surgery and gene therapy, is challenging. It should be made clean, that these may be first theoretical research procedures which may or may not help the fetus (*see* Fig 3.1A).

When there is a reasonable possibility that the fetal condition could be treated postnatally; there seems no justification for in-utero procedures.

ETHICAL ISSUES

It is not possible to address all the ethical issues associated with prenatal diagnosis, preimplantation diagnosis, fetal therapy and malignant pelvic masses in this chapter.

One of the most significant ethical issue is for a physician to offer a new invasive technique, with a relatively high/unknown risk to the patient. The burden of responsibility should not be shifted to the patient even if he/she gives informed consent for the same.

It may be further, argued that, the very offering of a procedure to a patient by a physician is a reasonable choice, and it was not a reasonable choice for the patient the physician would not have offered the same. Proper preliminary investigations in pregnancies destined for termination, must be appropriate patient selection followed by a fully informed consent would appear the most critical elements in satisfying the physician's ethical obligation in this regard.

It is, further, worthwhile to perform the invasive procedures on human recipients and collect the long-term benefit data, before applying it generally.

The initial human recipients should be informed that there is no information regarding the long-term consequences of these procedures in the patients or the children born subsequently.

Prenatal Diagnosis

An ethical dilemma, has arisen with prenatal diagnosis, as most of the couples can use this for sex-selection unrelated to the existence of X-linked disease. The other ethical issues arise are the increase risk of female feticide and also selection of normal human traits that is, designer babies.

Such procedures must only be advocated for diagnoses of genetic or pathological disorders. The distinction between normal variations and conditions like Down's syndrome and spina bifida seems apparent but the lines begin to blur when milder conditions also get diagnosed.

The other ethical issues are prenatal diagnosis of albinism, late onset Alzheimer's disease or familial hyper cholesterolemia should be addressed or not.

Another ethical dilemma arises in patients undergoing in vitro fertilization, where preimplantation diagnosis of embryos may be done and sex selection can be offered to the couple.

Abortion

The most important ethical dilemma today; is the ethics of selective abortion. These abortions of prenatal diagnosis should not be sex-selected procedures.

In case there is a genetic or fetal anomaly, then in an era of legalized abortions, the counsellor in an nondirective approach suggest to the couple the risk/benefits of abortion of the fetus in an individual case. Preferably, the physician may not be obligated in participating in the procedure and is best to refer the patient to an appropriate facility.

Furthermore, continuation of pregnancy in the face of a fetal abnormality, even a lethal one, must be presented as a valid alternative.

The physician must only recommend an abortion to the couple, in circumstances where there is a clear risk to the life or health of the mother.

The decision of the mother as regards to go for an abortion or not should be independently her own.

The Indian MTP Law is being amended to allow termination till 24 weeks.

Multiple Gestation

Complex and unique ethical dilemma may arise in a patient with multiple gestation, who is carrying both normal and abnormal fetuses.

Selective termination of the abnormal fetus can be offered to the patient, but is associated with a higher risk to the mother and the other normal fetus, than is associated with termination of a singleton pregnancy.

Therefore, the decision of selective feticide must be done taking all the pros and cons.

In case the fetus is suffering from a lethal condition (anencephaly or bilateral renal agenesis), it would be inappropriate to place the normal twin at an increased risk, provided the patient wants to continue the pregnancy. In the case of nonlethal but serious malformations (Down's syndrome or spina bifida), the patient must weigh the increased risk associated with a selective termination attempt of losing the normal twin against her wish not to give birth to the affected twin.

Ethical issues also present with selective feticide normal fetuses in multifetal gestation. This typically follows treatment for infertility and the goal is typically to improve the survival for the remaining living fetuses. It is also advocated that ethically some parents go for these procedures because they opt only for one child.

LEGAL ISSUES

It is not possible to provide a comprehensive discussion of the legal issues related to interventional procedures as there are no clear cut laws laid down. Currently to terminate pregnancy of over 20 weeks, legal permission from court is needed (MTP Law).

MEDICAL MALPRACTICE

The field of obstetrics and gynecology is under intense legal scrutiny and a large number of law suits have been filed. Generally speaking to prevail in a malpractice lawsuit a plaintiff must demonstrate that the physician breached the standard of care and this action or inaction caused injury.

Prenatal Diagnosis

Most malpractice laws suits involve failure to obtain an adequate family history or other relevant information leading to failure to identify factors that place the patient at increased risk of a specific birth defect or genetic disorder; failure to arrive at an accurate diagnoses.

In a patient who presents with findings that could reasonably lead to a diagnosis; failure to provide accurate genetic counseling; failure to offer prenatal diagnosis to patients at increased risk of having a child with a detectable disorder.

Another common allegation is failure to successfully informed consent prior to a diagnostic procedure.

Negligence in Performance of Interventional Ultrasound Techniques

The second category of allegations are in performance of an interventional procedure causing damage to the patient.

The patient has a legal right to expect the procedures will be performed using proper equipment by the skilled operator.

It is difficult to distinguish between a complication caused due to inherent risk of the procedure or from negligence. It is imperative, that the patient be counseled in advance of all complications that may occur.

Misdiagnosis

The final category of lawsuits involve allegations of error resulting in misdiagnosis or no diagnosis. These errors occur within the laboratory or inappropriate handling of the samples before they reach the laboratory.

It also includes, failure to identify a significant abnormality on ultrasound or diagnosis of an abnormality not actually present.

FETAL RESEARCH

Though a number of states have laws restricting fetal research, but the legal complexities related to the status of the embryo affect not only pre-implantation genetic diagnosis but also in vitro fertilization in general.

ABORTION

In India the upper legal age of abortion is 20 weeks but in case of malformed/congenitally there is no age limit.

CHAPTER 4

Interventional Ultrasound in Daily Obstetrical-Gynecological Practice

INTRODUCTION

The bimanual examination is still the main stay of the gynecological examination especially in resource poor settings; but even with experienced hands it can only furnish a limited assessment of pelvic structures.

Ultrasonography has improved the gynecological examination by adding an objective component, giving an insight into the precise size, internal appearance and structures of pelvic organs. It is also beneficial in patients with profuse vaginal bleeding, chronic medical conditions, children and girls who have not experienced intercourse.

We will discuss the different applications of office ultrasonography as related to invasive procedures done by gynecologist.

THE UTERINE CAVITY

Intrauterine Device

Most common indications of USG in this respect are:
- Confirm proper insertion of IUD
- Localize the IUD in case of "missing thread" within or outside the uterus

- Evaluate the cause of pain and bleeding in these patients.
- Myometrial invasion of IUD can be diagnosed when it extends beyond endometrium
- Correct positioning of IUD is measured on the longitudinal scan if the fundal distance is no more than 1/3rd greater than the thickness of the anterior and posterior uterine wall
- In difficult IUD extractions, USG helps in complete removal of device.

Minor Uterine Surgery

- USG helps in assisting in performance of intrauterine surgical procedures like curettage, excision of polyps and intracavitory fibroid; correct localization of instruments inside the uterine cavity
- It also helps in determining the completeness of a MTP, and D&C by showing an empty uterine cavity.

Postpartum Uterine Evaluation

Useful in case of PPH to diagnose retained bits of placenta and an USG guided D&C will reduce the chances of perforation and perform a compete procedure.

Sonohysterography [Saline Infusion Sonography (SIS)]

It is a fluid enhanced TVS which can distinguish between intracavitory tissue and polyp or fibroids.

Ultrasound-guided Prenatal Diagnostic Procedures

Chorion villus sampling, amniocentesis and fetal blood sampling can establish the presence of fetal disease.

THE FALLOPIAN TUBE

Color flow sonosalpingography and 3D contrast sonosalpingography is used to determine tubal patency and uterine cavity.

USG guided transcervical tubal catheterization can be performed in ambulatory settings and is fast replacing the more invasive procedures (abdominal and laparoscopic surgery). It is also enhancing IVF fertilization in patients with tubal occlusion.

This technique not only diagnoses the tubal disease but is also employed in treatment of tubal occlusion by transcervical balloon tuboplasty with fluoroscopy and ultrasonography.

Permanent Contraception

Transcervical tubal catheterization can be used to occlude the tubes by cryocoagulation, electrocoagulation silicone plugs and chemical injection, but all are associated with high failure rates.

Assisted Reproduction

USG guided tubal catheterization can be performed for tubal placement of embryos and gametes is a simple procedure and there is no radiation risk.

Ectopic Pregnancy

In early detected ectopic pregnancies by TVS, local deposition of cytodestructive agents (methotrexate) may reduce the amount of medication delivered and its serious systemic side effects.

THE CERVIX

Cervical incompetence is the inability of the uterus to maintain a pregnancy until term due to cervical defect—congenital or acquired due to trauma, cone biopsy or tumors.

The cervical length and internal os diameter can be effectively measured by ultrasonography especially TVS. So, the most important predictor of preterm birth before 30 weeks gestation was an internal os diameter of 5 mm or more and cervical length of less than 2 cms.

Cervical effacement starts at the level of internal os and can be easily detected by TVS and prevent measures to prevent abortion or preterm labor can be taken by complete bed rest, to uterine relaxants and cervical encirclage preferably at 13-14 weeks of gestation.

USG is employed to guide the placement of suture and determine if the internal os is closed effectively and good cervical length is achieved or not.

USG is advantageous in providing the exact location of internal os, location of membranes, decreased risk of puncturing the amniotic sac and visualization of actual closure of the cervix after placement of the suture and follow-up.

CHAPTER 5

Obstetric Procedures—Overview

COUNSELING AND PATIENT PREPARATIONS

- Obstetric interventional procedures are usually performed for diagnosis and therapy
- Diagnostic obstetric procedures are for prenatal diagnosis in patients identified to be at a risk of birth defects or genetic defects
- Therapeutic obstetric procedures are an attempt to give some palliative treatment intrauterine so as to save the fetus from damage/death until a gestation of viability.

For counseling one needs to observe the following points:
- Communication with the patient and family
- Explain medical facts, diagnosis, probable cause of disorder and options of management
- Heredity
- Risk of recurrence
- Course of action and options
- Ethical, religious and social counseling
- Explain procedural risks and side effects and complications.
- Discussion of ethical dilemmas of procedure benefit and balance of procedure related risks
- Choice of abortion

- Choice of fetal reduction in high order multiple gestations
- Misdiagnosis and limitations (Not all misdiagnosis are due to negligence)
- Risk stratification by screening test (Refer to Flowchart 1.1A).

TRICKS OF INTERVENTIONAL ULTRASOUND

A sound knowledge of the following:
- *Physics of ultrasound*: It is essential for the sonologist to be aware of the working of ultrasound machines and the way images are generated and how the resolution can be improved
- *Artefact*: It is essential to understand reverberation artefacts and comet tail artefacts, mirror image artifacts. Chinese hat artifact, etc. otherwise many procedures will be not done or done incorrectly
- *Invasive procedures*: To do invasive procedures the operator must be well versed with using correct transducer, correct instruments, proper gain controls
  The common obstetric procedures will be:
    - CVS
    - Amniocentesis
    - Cord blood sampling
    - Fetal biopsy (Figs. 5.1 to 5.4)
    - Fetal blood transfusion
    - Fetal shunts
    - Twin gestation for TRAP syndrome.
- *Technical aspects*: Freehand or biopsy guide technique. Angle of needle in freehand technique should be 90° to the beam. Single operator or two operator technique. Use of sono enhanced needles

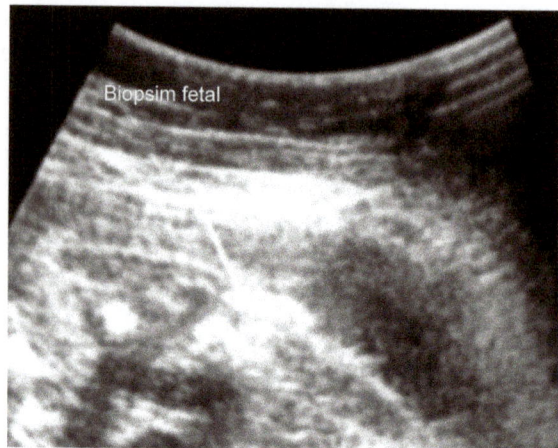

Fig. 5.1: Biopsy of the fetal muscle.

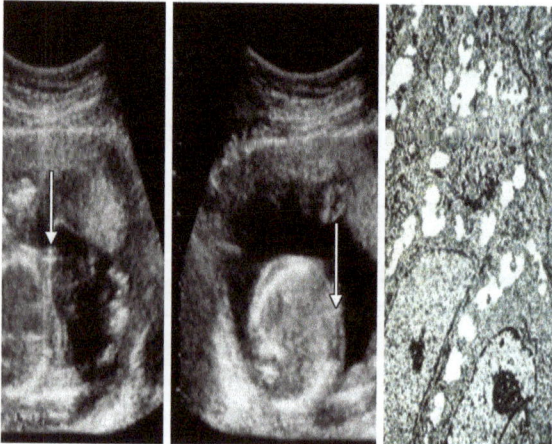

Fig. 5.2: Biopsy of the fetal skin.

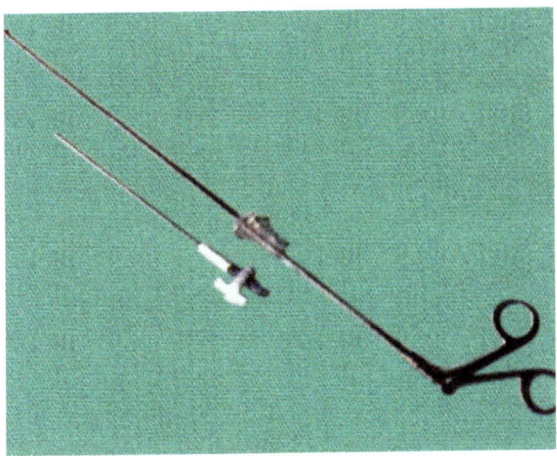

Fig. 5.3: Needles for biopsy of the fetal skin.

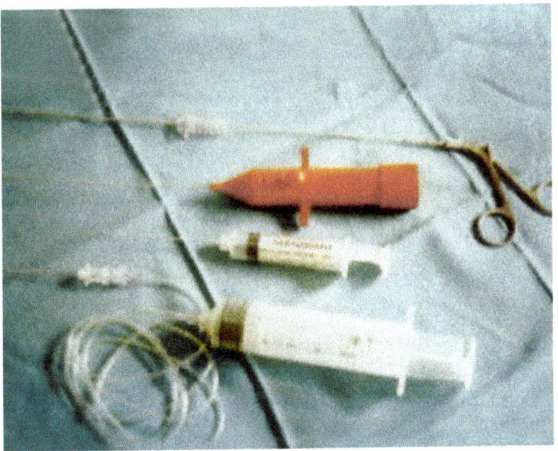

Fig. 5.4: Instruments for biopsy of the fetal skin.

PROCEDURES

All invasive obstetric procedures are aimed at making a prenatal diagnosis in patients at risk of congenital genetic malformations, a few of these procedures are also aimed at therapeutically saving the fetus *in utero* till the time of viability when they can be delivered for further pediatric surgical management.

ANESTHESIA AND PLACE

As discussed earlier all obstetric interventional procedures should be done in:
- Hospital OT
- Minor OT set-up
- Under analgesia, local anesthesia
- Short general anesthesia
- Proper informed consent with pre and post test counceling.

CHORIONIC VILLOUS SAMPLING (FIGS. 5.5 TO 5.10)

- First trimester modality
- Aims to retrieve adequate trophoblastic tissue
- USG guided procedure
- TAS and transcervical CVS
- TVS and transmyometrial CVS
- TAS and free hand/biopsy abdominal CVS
- CVS needle (malleable)
- TAS with partially full bladder to identify chorionic tissue
- Lithotomy position
- Asepsis and vaginal cleaning
- Hold anterior lip of cervix
- Guide the CVS needle gently towards lower end of implantation site under direct vision

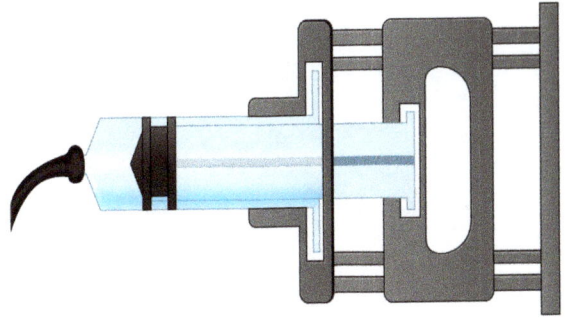

Fig. 5.5: Syringe used for an abdominal CVS.

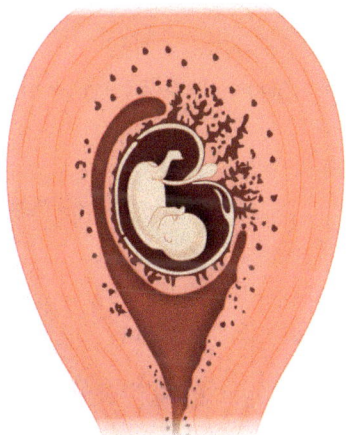

Fig. 5.6: A schematic diagram of the chorion to delineate the site for CVS.

- Suction with a 5 cc syringe and very gentle curetting movements
- Tissue retrieved and send in culture media for karyotyping and culture
- Transabdominal sampling done by single or double needle technique

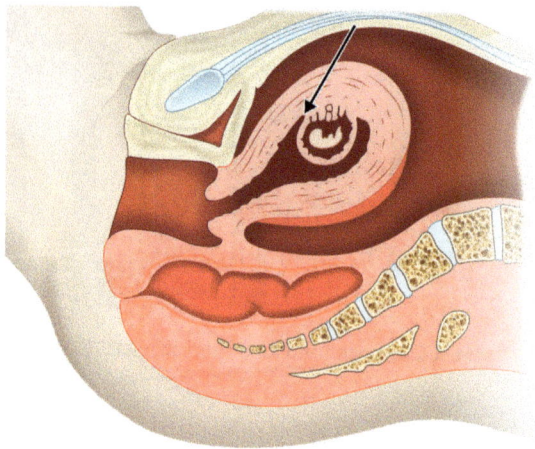

Fig. 5.7: Schematic diagram of a CVS being done transabdominally.

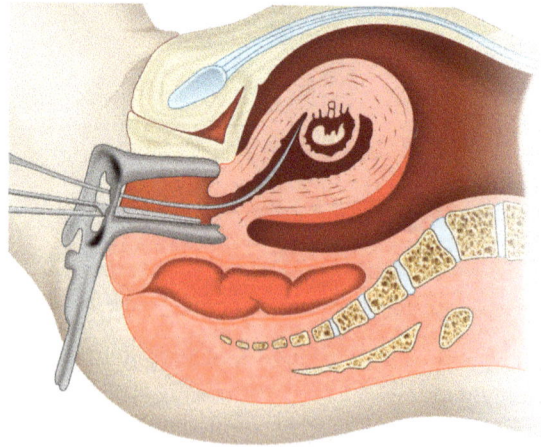

Fig. 5.8: Schematic diagram of a CVS being done transvaginally.

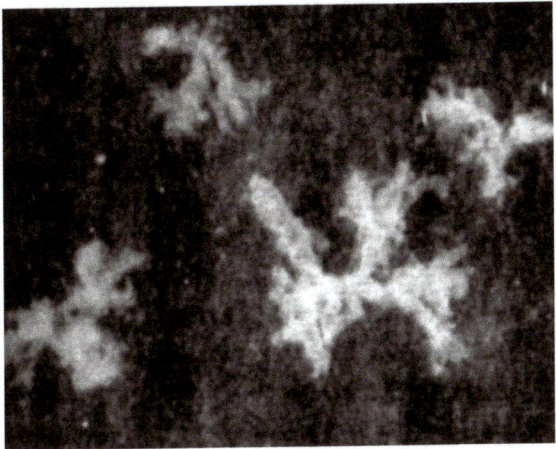

Fig. 5.9: Villi as seen in the Petri dish after the procedure.

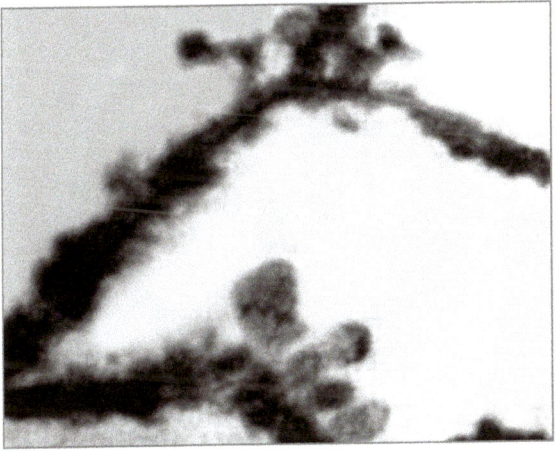

Fig. 5.10: Villi as seen through a microscope.

- Ideal time 9–12 weeks
- Counseling of patient for pregnancy loss and genetic disorders
- *Side effects*: Pregnancy loss, bleeding, failure to retrieve tissue, rupture of membranes, infection, elevated MSAFP, Rh isoimmunization, limb body anomalies.

AMNIOCENTESIS AND COELOCENTESIS (FIGS. 5.11 TO 5.14)

Coelocentesis

- Coelomic aspiration under USG guidance
- TVS scan to locate anatomy
- No anesthesia or only mild sedation
- 20 gauge needle through a biopsy guide/transmyometrial

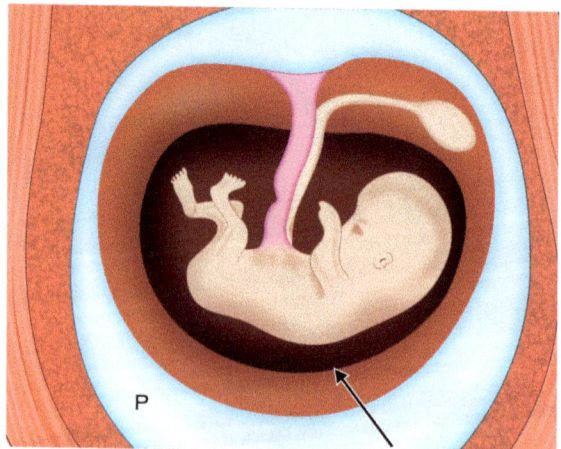

Fig. 5.11: Schematic diagram of coelocentesis.

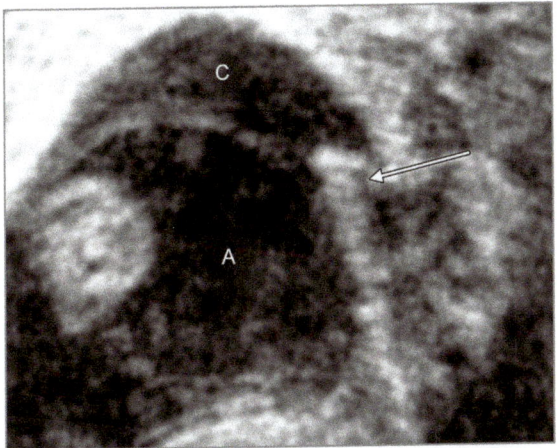

Fig. 5.12: Placement of the needle (coelocentesis).

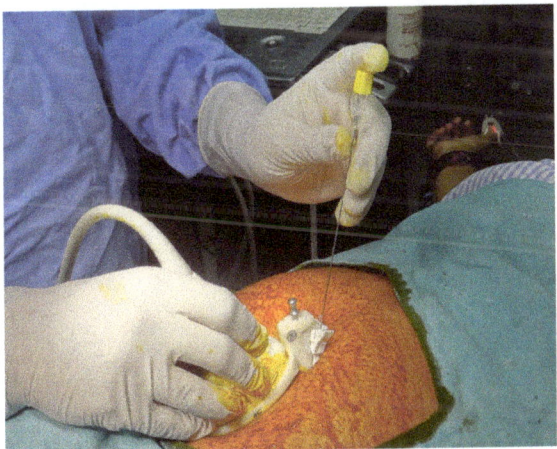

Fig. 5.13: Freehand technique for amniocentesis (II).

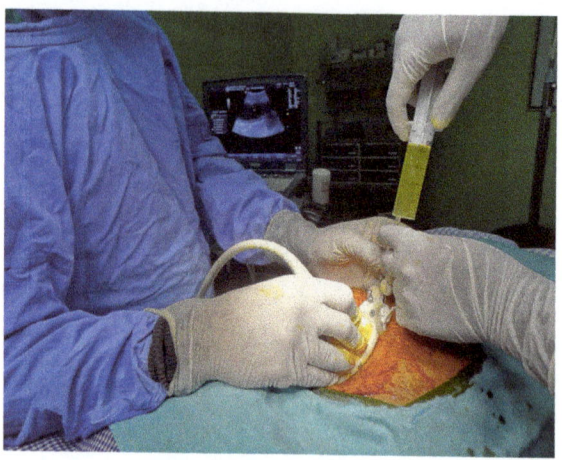

Fig. 5.14: Freehand technique for amniocentesis (I).

- Needle placed in coelomic cavity
- Fluid is aspirated (0.5–2.5 mL).

Amniocentesis (17 Weeks Onwards)

- Indications
    - Cytogenetic diagnosis
    - NTD: Late first or early second trimester
    - Metabolic defects
    - Isoimmunization
    - Fetal lung maturity
    - Late second or early third trimester
    - Intra-amniotic infection
    - PROM
    - Drainage of polyhydramnios
    - Medical treatment of fetus
    - Therapeutic.

- Selection of a needle (18–22 gauge spinal needle)
- USG scan to identify pocket free of placenta and cord and fetal parts
- Ultrasonographically guided amniocentesis
- Ultrasonographically monitored amniocentesis
- Convex probe or sector probe or even linear probe is TAS (Figs. 5.13 and 5.14)
- Needle with stylet introduced by freehand technique or fixed biopsy guide technique
- Stylet removed and amniotic fluid aspirated
- 0.5 mL first fluid is discarded to avoid maternal cell contamination
- 5–15 mL fluid is aspirated and sent for karyotyping of fetal cells and for genetic culture.

Early Amniocentesis

- Procedure before 15 weeks gestation
- Equal diagnostic potential as a mid-trimester amniocentesis with added advantage of an easier termination if required
- Can be done TVS guided also.

Complications

- Fetal loss
- Fetal injury
- Fetal respiratory complication (Macaca fasicularis)
- Amniotic fluid leakage
- Bloody taps
- Fetomaternal transfusion
- Infection
- Meconium staining
- Rh isoimmunization.

CORD BLOOD SAMPLING (CORDOCENTESIS) (FIGS. 5.15 TO 5.21)

With the development of interventional ultrasound in obstetrics an access to fetal circulation was discovered. Access to fetal blood and fetal circulation has led to our improvement of many fetal diseases, diagnosis and diagnosis of fetal acidemia and even therapy. Fetal blood sample provides fetal lymphocytes through which faster and more accurate genetic diagnosis can be made.

Indications

- Cytogenetics
- Viral and parasitic infections
- Red blood cell alloimmunization
- Fetal thrombocytopenia
- Nonimmune hydrops evaluation

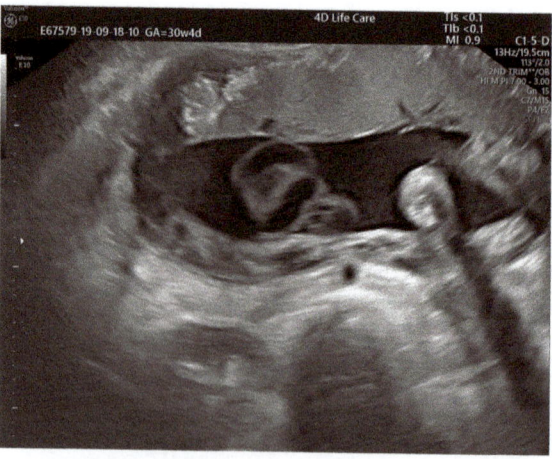

Fig. 5.15: Free loop of umbilical cord seen on a 2D scan.

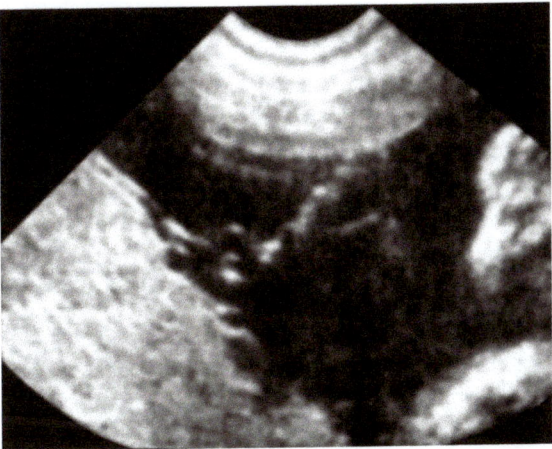

Fig. 5.16: Definitely see that you look for a free loop of umbilical cord.

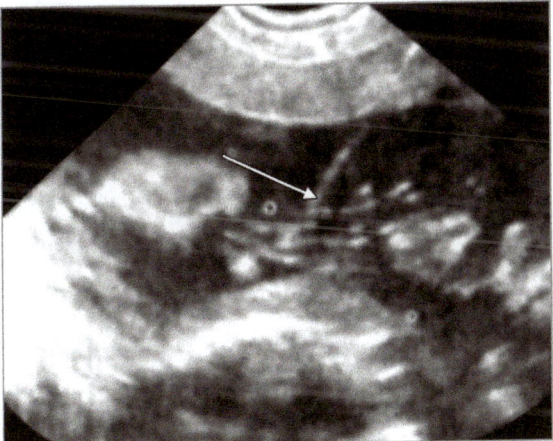

Fig. 5.17: Arrow showing the placement of the needle.

44 Interventional Ultrasound in Obstetrics and Gynecology

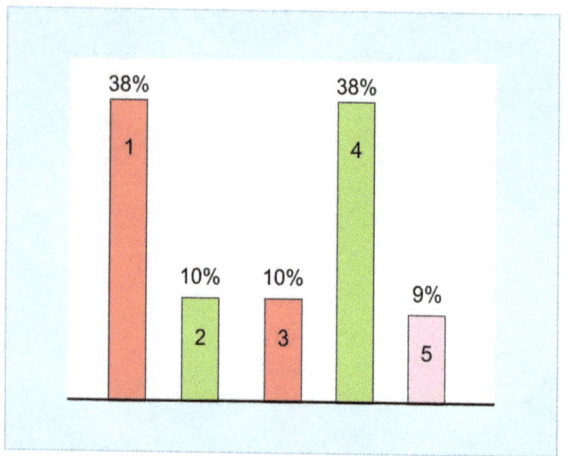

Fig. 5.18: Routes for cordocentesis depending on the free loop and the site of the placenta.

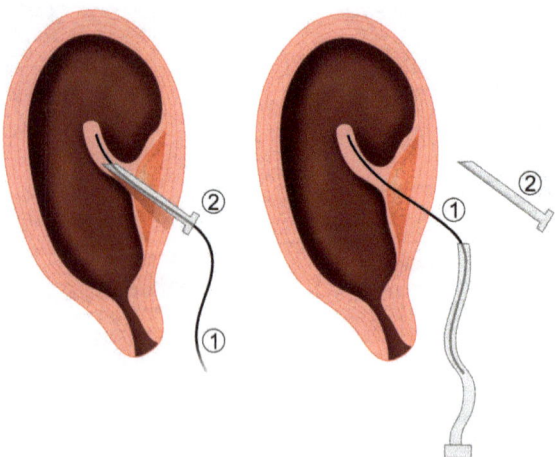

Fig. 5.19: Catheterization of the umbilical cord.

Obstetric Procedures—Overview

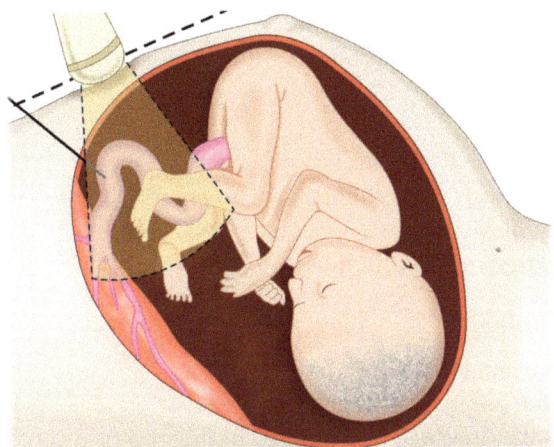

Fig. 5.20: Transducer position, fetal position and the technique for cordocentesis.

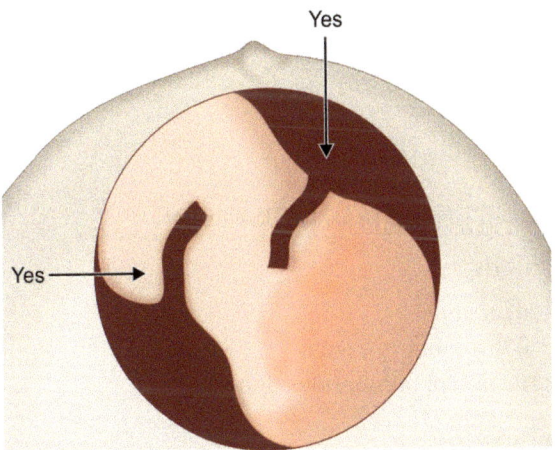

Fig. 5.21: Proper technique and route for cordocentesis.

- Perinatal fetal assessment
- Twin-twin transfusion and TRAP evaluation.

Sites

- Free loop of umbilical cord (Loop)
- Umbilical fetal abdomen attachment (Fetal abdomen)
- Umbilical placental attachment (Placenta)
- Fetal portal vein (intrahepatic) (Portal vein).

Technique

- Free hand (*See* Fig. 5.13)
- Fixed biopsy guide
- 20–22 gauge needle (spinal)
- Local anesthesia and strict asepsis
- 2–5 mL blood in dry heparinized syringes.

Complications

- Failure to obtain blood or contaminated blood (maternal)
- Fetal loss
- Infection
- Amniotic fluid loss.

INTRAUTERINE FETAL TRANSFUSION

Indications

- Fetal anemia
- Fetal thrombocytopenia
- Correction of immunodeficiencies.

Technique

- Intravascular (in umbilical vein)
- Intraperitoneally (in fetus).

Intravascular transfusion can be given in the umbilical vein free loop, intrahepatic portion or even exceptionally in left cardiac ventricle. Interperitoneal transfusion may be performed from 14 weeks gestation.

- 20 gauge spinal needle
- Bolus transfusion or an intrauterine exchange can be given via a 3 way valve.

Risks and Complications

- Procedure related risk
- Transfusion risk
- Alloimmunization risk.

FETAL SHUNTS (FIG. 5.22)

Fetal shunting should be contemplated for conditions frequently associated with significant neonatal mortality and morbidity.

Indications

- Obstructive uropathy
- Pleural effusion
- Pulmonary cysts
- Ventriculomegaly
- Fetal ascites.

Fetal Invasive Therapy

- Natural history of condition should be known
- Condition severe enough to interfere with normal development and cause death or disability
- Treatment should be capable of improving the natural history of the condition
- Evidence from animal models should support this

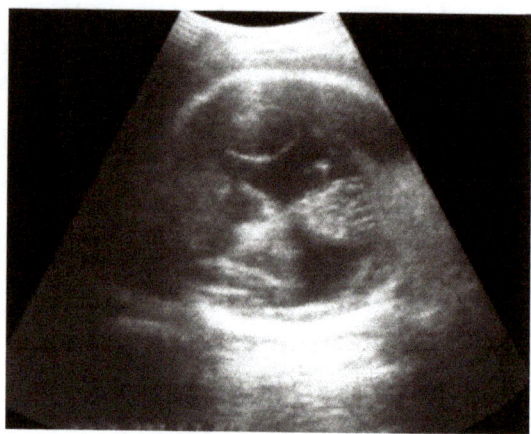

Fig. 5.22: Hydrocephalus puncture for termination.

- Exclude all other fetal anomalies
- Reliable prognostic tests
- Immature fetus for delivery
- Benefits to fetus must outweigh risks
- Counseling and informed consent
- Proper ANC and follow-up
- Postnatal corrective methods
- Scientifically evaluated treatment.

Types of Shunt

1. Vesico-amniotic : Obstructive uropathy
   Posterior urethral valve
2. Pyleo-amniotic : Hydronephrosis
3. Pleuro-amniotic : Hydrothorax/chylothorax
4. Cysto-amniotic : Pulmonary cyst
5. Peritoneo-amniotic : Ascites
6. Ventriculo-amniotic : Cerebral ventriculomegaly

Technique

- Skilled personnel
- Genetic treatment centers (quaternary referral)
- Written consent
- Counseling
- OPD procedure
- Mild analgesia/anesthesia
- Fetal injection pancuronium (to paralyze fetus: temporary)
- Prophylactic antibiotics.

Types of Shunts

Rocket fetal catheter: A double pigtail silastic catheter (external and internal diameter 2.1 and 5.1 mm)

- High resolution scan to identify target
- Asepsis
- 20 gauge spinal needle in amniotic cavity and amnio-infusion with 150–200 mL warm saline
- Introduction of metal trocar in target site and drainage of target fluid
- Fetal catheter is straightened and introduced
- Withdrawal of cannula.

The procedure of shunts is not without risks and maternal and fetal complications.

Today great advances have taken place in form of microendoscope and laser techniques to deal with such cases.

INTRAUTERINE PRESSURE ASSESSMENT (FIG. 5.23)

Intra-amniotic pressures are studied in labour and in conditions of poly and oligohydramnios and in fetal body cavities.

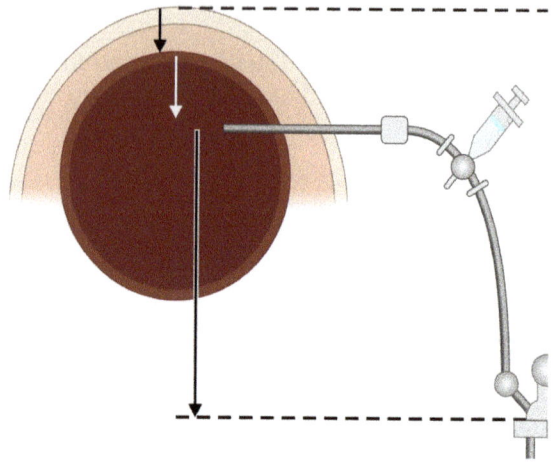

Fig. 5.23: Intra-amniotic pressure assessment.

Pressure changes equipment are available, a needle is passed into the cavity of whose pressure has to be evaluated and connected to the pressure detection system.

In the last 10 years many studies have been reported of intrauterine and intrafetal pressures and their importance in antenatal surveillance. These help in understanding fetal pathophysiology but at the current status are a research tool.

DIAGNOSTIC AND THERAPEUTIC MEASURES IN TWINS (FIGS. 5.24 TO 5.26)

All procedures done in singleton pregnancies for prenatal diagnosis can be done in twins also (amniocentesis, CVS, cord blood sampling, etc.). In monochorionic twins special procedures can be done to improve outcome.

Obstetric Procedures—Overview

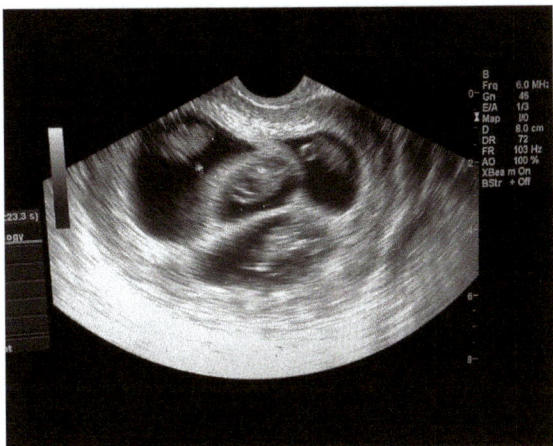

Fig. 5.24: Multifetal pregnancy for reduction.

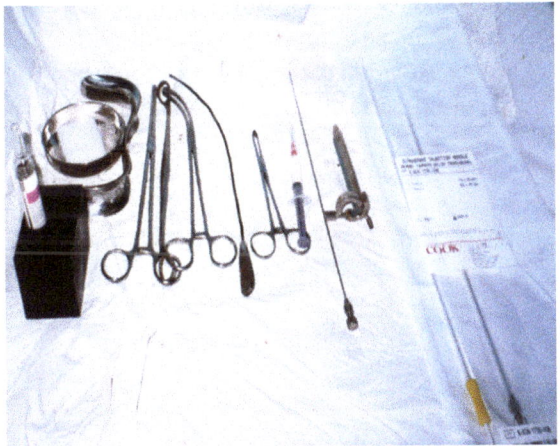

Fig. 5.25: Equipment for fetal reduction.

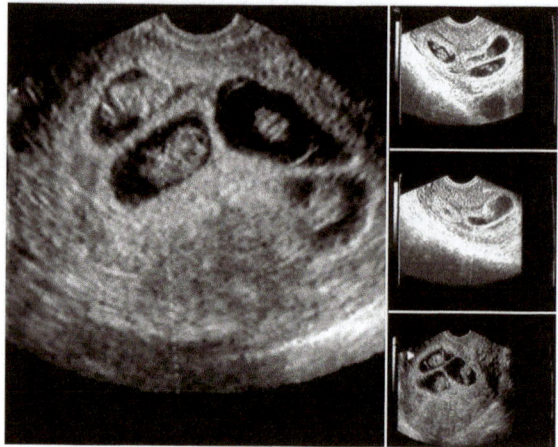

Fig. 5.26: Stepwise reduction of two fetuses in a quadruplet pregnancy.

- Twin to twin transfusion syndrome
  - Amniodrainage by an 18 gauge needle
  - Laser coagulation of placental anastomosis
  - Selective feticide of acardiac twin in TRAP syndrome.

CHAPTER 6

Anesthesia for Interventional Ultrasound in Obstetrics

Ultrasound is an important tool to make early diagnosis of fetal lesions which can be treated percutaneously during pregnancy.

Most of the treatments require anesthesia because, due to maternal anxiety there is rise of catecholamines which may compromise the fetus by lowering placental blood flow and predisposing to preterm labor.

In order to limits these events anesthesia is required which is a little different due to the physiological changes, that occur during pregnancy.

PHYSIOLOGICAL CHANGES OF PREGNANCY

Many of the maternal physiological changes can influence this conduct of anesthesia.

Cardiovascular System

The maternal cardiac output at term increases by 30–40%, plasma volume by 50%, red cell mass by 30%. The systemic vascular resistance is reduced.

Autocaval compression becomes clinical significant in supine position after 10 weeks of gestation, reducing venous return (VR), cardiac output (CO) and uteroplacental perfusion.

Inferior vena caval compression due to the gravid uterus is associated with venous stasis and increase chances of thrombophlebitis.

Alterations in many coagulation factor (increase in factor VIII, XII and fibrinogen and decrease in factor XI, XIII) may potentiate the risk of venous thrombosis.

Respiratory Function

Minute alveolar ventilation increases during pregnancy leading to respiratory alkalosis, which is compensated by two kidneys by renal excretion of bicarbonate in order to maintain normal acid-base balance.

Pregnancy creates a decreased ability to buffer an acidotic state. While maternal oxygen consumption increases, functional residual capacity decreases so hypoxia occurs rapidly.

Gastrointestinal Tract

As the uterus expands, the maternal stomach is shifted cephalad and in a horizontal posterior, altering the gastroesophageal angle, reducing the competency of esophageal sphincter. Simultaneously, the gastric acid production increases.

Both these factors predispose to passive regurgitation and more chances of aspiration of gastric contents during general anesthesia.

ANESTHETIC DRUGS

The increase in cardiac output, glomerular filtration and volume of distribution and decrease in plasma proteins alters the pharmokinetics of anesthetic agents.

Secondly, due to hormonal changes, pregnant women are more sensitive to the effects of general and local anesthetic agents.

These drugs may also cross the placental barrier and affect the fetus. Furthermore, some anesthetic agents are teratogenic too.

Spinal/Regional anesthesia when appropriate minimizes fetal drug exposure and is safer.

Anesthetic drugs effect the meternal and these drugs may also affect the fetus indirectly by altering the uterine flow and/or placental blood flow.

ANESTHETIC TECHNIQUES

Positioning

Left uterine tilt is essential to avoid aortocaval compression and ensure optimal uterine blood flow.

Monitoring

Intraoperative monitoring consists of pulse oximetry, non-invasive blood pressure estimation, electrocardiographic display, fetal heart rate and uterine activity is monitored throughout the procedure.

Preoperative Period

Preanesthetic check-up and proper counseling regarding the risks of anesthesia are to be taken prior to the procedure and written informed consent is to be taken.

Systemic preoperative screenings are not mandatory but can be done. A coagulation profile and electrocardiogram are also justified.

Premedication with benzodiazepine to allay anxiety of mother, per rectal indomethacin to prevent preterm labor and antacid with antiemetic combination is given to prevent gastric acid aspiration.

Local and Regional Anesthesia

For percutaneous procedures, local anesthesia by skin infilteration is used as it easy, safe and avoids risk of maternal aspiration associated with general anesthesia. All local anesthetic agents cross the placental barrier and may depress the fetal cardiovascular system, so they must be infused into the general circulation. The use of large size needles and multiple punctures may cause catecholamine secretion causing increase uterine arterial resistance, lowering placental blood flow and uncoordinated uterine contractions and preterm labor.

Although spinal/epidural anesthesia is safe for the mother but may cause a fall in blood pressure, decrease in uterine blood flow and increased risk of fetal hypoxia. Early detection of maternal hypotension and early correction with vascular fluid loading and ephedrine is advised.

Neither local/regional anesthesia administered to the mother provide anesthesia to the fetus.

Fetal anesthesia can be attained by administration of mother with benzodiazepines and opiates, but these drugs can depress maternal ventilation and cause fetal hypoxemia, acidosis and cardiac depression.

Hypercarbia also causes maternal catecholamine seretion leading to reduction uterine blood flow.

General Anesthesia

This allows more accurate control of maternal ventilation. blood pressure and also provides adequate fetal anesthesia.

Induction

The usual "full stomach" precaution has to be taken. Maternally administered anesthetics have indirect effect on the fetus due to maternal hypotension and release of catecholamines during airway instrumentation.

Maintenance

Nitrous oxide in oxygen and halogenated agents provide adequate maternal relaxation and fetal anesthesia. The halogenated anesthetic agents may cause hypotension and is further worsened by increased uterine blood flow due to uterine relaxation.

Intraoperative narcotics and benzodiazepine are used to reduce maternal adrenergic response to surgical stimulation that are deleterious for placental blood flow.

Narcotics given to mother will produce fetal analgesia and lack of movements. Benzodiazepines cause fetal amnesia which may decrease fetal response to subsequent stressful stimuli.

Fetal immobility is also caused due to muscle relaxation and reversal of neuromuscular blockade with anticholinesterase can increase uterine muscle tone.

Uterine relaxation is important for both operative comfort and placental blood flow and can be obtained by halogenated agents like halothane etc. These agents lower uterine vascular resistance and maintain uteroplacental blood flow.

It is also important that a pregnant woman maintains normocarbia.

Hyperventilation and resulting hypocarbia produces vasoconstriction and decreases uterine blood flow. Secondly, it also causes respiratory alkalosis causing a leftward shift of the hemoglobin dissociation curve and decrease in oxygen availability for the fetus.

Hypercarbia due to hypoventilation raises the maternal catecholamine concentration resulting in reduced uterine blood flow.

Postoperative Period

Tocolytics must be used with strict monitoring of the maternal electrocardiogram. Continuous fetal and uterine activity monitoring must be done decreasing the whole postoperative period. Adequate pain relief must be given to the mother as it decreases maternal plasma catecholamines and help prevent the onset of premature labor.

CHAPTER 7

Ultrasound-guided Techniques in Fetal Medicine

INTRODUCTION

All ultrasound-guided diagnostic and therapeutic invasive procedures in fetal medicine are best done transabdominally by essentially using the same technique; which ensure minimization of risks with introduction of a new technique.

Another prerequisite for invasive procedures is that operator should have extensive experience in ultrasound scanning.

Invasive procedures are best performed by a curvilinear transducer as it combines the advantages of both linear array and sector systems, so the needle is visualized throughout its length and image of the tip is sharp.

A free-hand technique is preferred as it allows freedom for manipulation especially if the posterior of the target is suddenly altered by uterine contractions or fetal movements.

PROCEDURES

- A detailed ultrasound is performed to define the position of fetus, placenta and adnexal vessels/masses
- A lateral entry into the uterus is preferred irrespective of the position of the placenta (anterior or posterior) as laterally the visualization and manipulation is easier (Fig. 7.1)

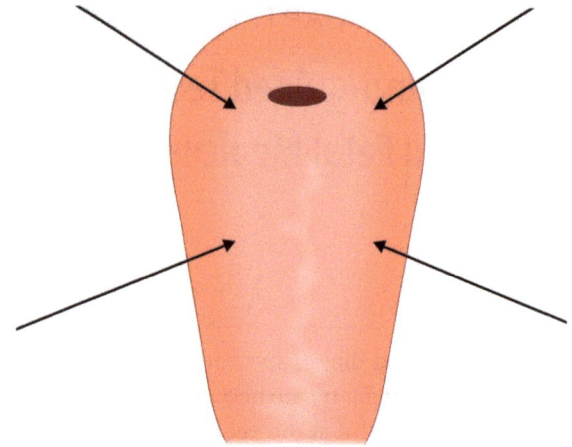

Fig. 7.1: Preferred entries to the uterus.

- Potential sites of skin puncture are from 1 o'clock to 5 o'clock on the left and 7 o'clock to 11 o'clock on the right
- The transducer is held in the left hand of a right-handed operator
- The desired target is identified and the transducer is aligned in such a way, that, the target lies in the center of the screen and the proposed site of entry on the maternal abdomen is visualized at the edge of the screen
- Starting from "five past seven position" the transducer which is always kept at right angles to the operating table, is gradually rotated for systematic examination of all potential sites of entry and identification of the most suitable one
- Place the right index finger on the maternal abdomen about 2-3 cm away from the edge of the transducer and pressed firmly toward the uterus (Fig. 7.2)

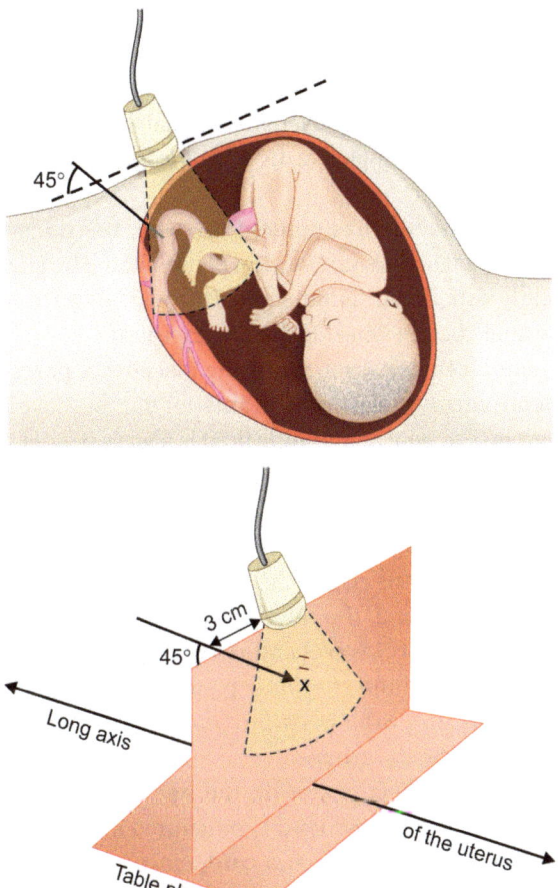

Fig. 7.2: Technique for ultrasound-guided procedures.

- When the transducer and finger are in the same plane, the indentation caused by the finger is clearly visible which helps the operator to simulate needle insertion

- The chosen site of entry is cleaned and dropped and local anesthesia is infiltrated (under ultrasound guidance)
- The needle/instrument is then introduced into the uterus, ensuring that the whole length is visualized continuously; with the needle angled at 45° from the horizontal plane of the transducer
- Once the needle has entered the skin, the transducer, maintained in the same vertical plane, should be angled to clearly visualize the initial shaft of the needle and to correct the angle before entering the myometrium
- In amniocentesis, even when the placenta is posterior, a lateral entry is preferred to an anterior one, because in this position the pool of amniotic fluid is always deeper
- For chorionic villus sampling even with a posterior placenta usually there is lateral extension of the placenta, so it becomes risky to enter the amniotic cavity
- For cordocentesis (Figs. 7.3A to C), when the placenta is anterior or lateral, the needle is passed transplacentally into the umbilical vessel and visualized longitudinally. It is best to avoid the chorionic plate and amniotic cavity, as puncturing the chorionic plate vessel can lead to catastrophic hemorrhage
- When placenta is posterior, the needle in introduced transamniotically and cord is punctured at right angle to the longitudinal axis of the cord, close to the placental insertion when fetal parts obscure the placental insertion appropriate external pressure may be needed to change the fetal position
- For fetal dermatocentesis, the needle is inserted at right angles to the longitudinal axis of the fetus and it is best to take skin biopsies from fetal buttocks or scalp

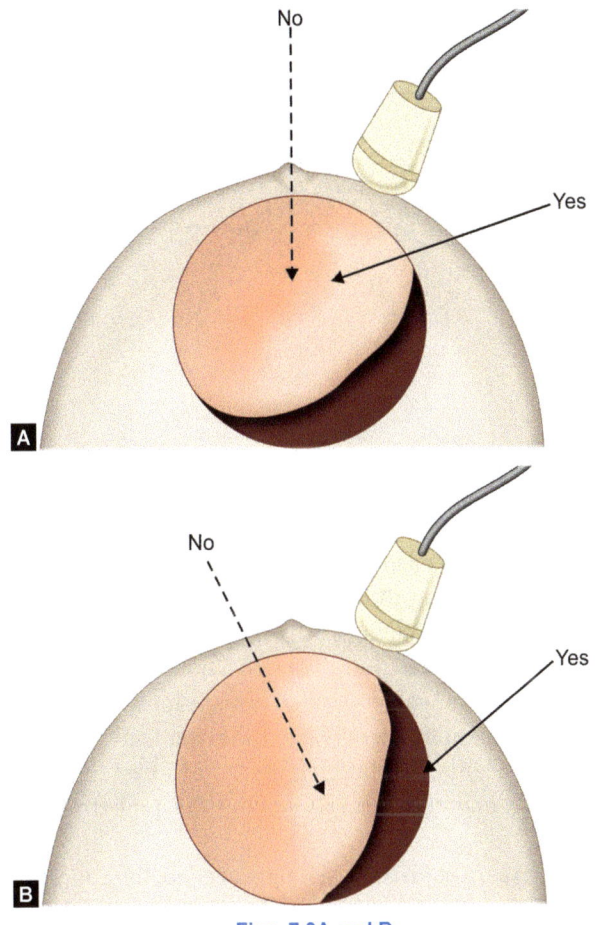

Figs. 7.3A and B

- For fetal hepatocentesis, the needle at right angles to the longitudinal axis of the fetal abdomen is directed to the right hypochondrium

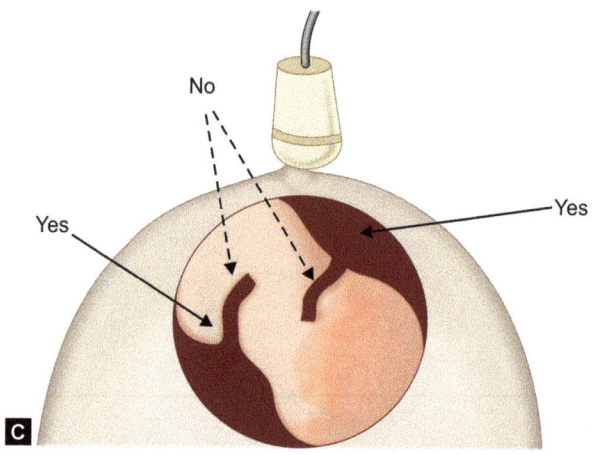

Figs. 7.3A to C: Cordocentesis.

- For fetal bladder aspiration (Urodochocentesis), of vesico-amniotic shunting, the needle cannula is introduced inferolaterally into the bladder at right angle to the fetal trunk, taking care to avoid puncturing the umbilicus
- For intraperitoneal fetal blood transfusions, the needle is introduced anterolaterally into the lower fetal abdomen.
- For thoracoamniotic shunting, the thorax is best approached posterolaterally (anterior shunts are often pulled out by the fetus)
- If drainage of contralateral lung is needed, the appropriate fetal position is achieved by rotating the fetal body using the tip of the cannula.

CHAPTER 8

Coelocentesis

INTRODUCTION

Coelomic fluid can be successfully aspirated by transvaginal puncture between 6 and 12 weeks of gestation and is less traumatic to fetus and early placenta as compared to early amniocentesis and chorionic villus sampling.

Endocoelomic cavity can be visualized at 6 weeks. Maximum size is attained at 9 weeks (5–6 mL).

TECHNIQUE

Coelomic aspiration is performed under ultrasonographic guidance using a high-frequency transvaginal probe. The vagina is cleaned with an antiseptic solution such as chlorhexamine glutamate 0.05% and cetrimide 0.5% to minimize the risk of a bacterial contamination. Transvaginal scan is performed to locate the fetus, amniotic membrane intraembryonic coelomic cavity and yolk sac. Anesthesia is not required.

A needle guide is attached to shaft of probe and a 20 gauge needle is introduced into the coelomic cavity under ultrasound scanning taking care to avoid puncture of amniotic membrane or yolk sac. The needle should be introduced into the uterus centrally through anterior wall to avoid injury to uterine vessels, chances of bowel puncture is also reduced and accidental bladder puncture is unlikely to be associated with significant complication; it is better avoided.

Needle should always be parallel to the amniotic membrane otherwise membrane tends to attach to the needle tip and abstruct coelomic fluid aspiration.

Needle should be placed as far as possible from yolk sac, to avoid injury to these mobile structures.

Endocoelomic fluid can be aspirated with 100% success rate between 6 and 10 weeks. Volume of fluid for diagnostic purpose is 0.5–2.5 mL. The color is yellow and is more viscous than amniotic fluid. This helps to recognize inadvertent puncture of amniotic cavity during coelocentesis.

Coelocentesis in Prenatal Diagnosis (Figs. 8.1 and 8.2)

- Ninety five precent success rate between >6 and 10 weeks of gestation

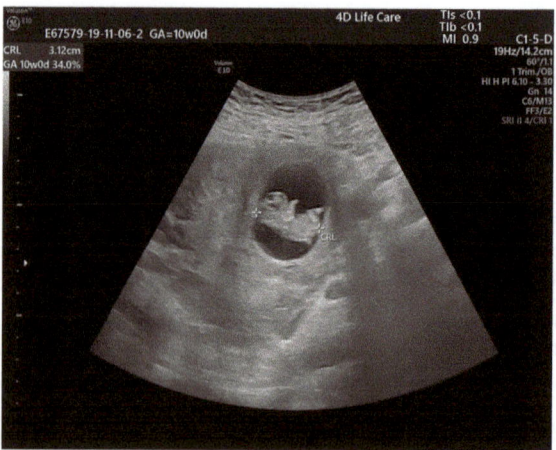

Fig. 8.1: Transvaginal ultrasonic view of the gestational sac at 10 weeks gestation.

- Risk of injury to growing embryo and placenta is less
- Easy to learn
- Minimal discomfort to mother
- Low rate of contamination of sample with maternal cells.

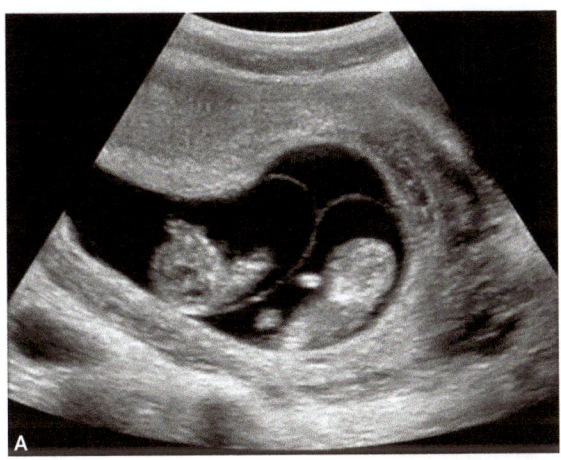

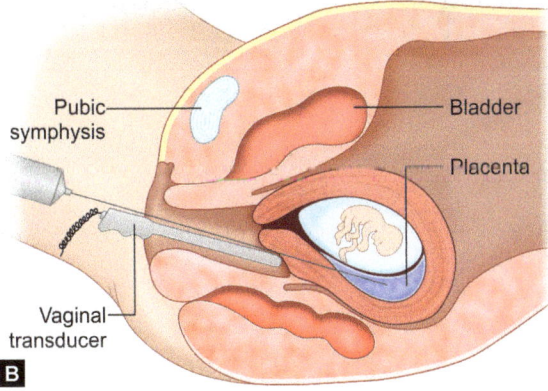

Figs. 8.2A and B: (A) Coelocentesis at 10 weeks' gestation.
(B) Schematic representation.

Coelomic fluid contain cells that are mostly hematopoietic in origin and predominantly erythroid lineage.

Ninety precent of cells are viable before 7 weeks. Between 8 and 10 weeks the viability, decreases to 30-50%. The viability of the cells is the primary determinant of cell culture success. The number of dividing cells in culture before 7 weeks gestation are sufficient for diagnostic purpose.

Diagnosis of sickle cell anemia and human single gene disorder is feasible by analysis of coelomic fluid in early pregnancy.

The feasibility of karyotyping by coelocentesis remain uncertain.

CHAPTER 9

Chorionic Villus Sampling

INTRODUCTION

It is a first trimester prenatal diagnostic test in which samples of chorionic villi are taken from chorion frondosum by an ultrasound guided catheter.

The ideal time for sampling is the 70–91st day from the last menstrual period because nuchal fold can be seen and measured. Chorion frondosum contains intricatively active villi and therefore preferred biopsy site.

CVS procedure should not be performed before 70th day after LMP.

- *Cervical culture*: For *Neisseria gonorrhoeae* to avoid chorioamnionitis
- *Genetic counseling*: Patient should be explained risk of procedure as well as limitations
- An ultrasound 1–3 weeks prior to anticipated date of procedure should be performed to evaluate fetal viability, gestation age, presence of twins, pregnancy related pathology chorionic hematoma or blighted ovum that could affect the procedure and its interpretation (Fig. 9.1)
- On day of sampling USG should be repeated to confirm continued viability and appropriate growth of embryo. Nuchal fold can be seen and should be measured.

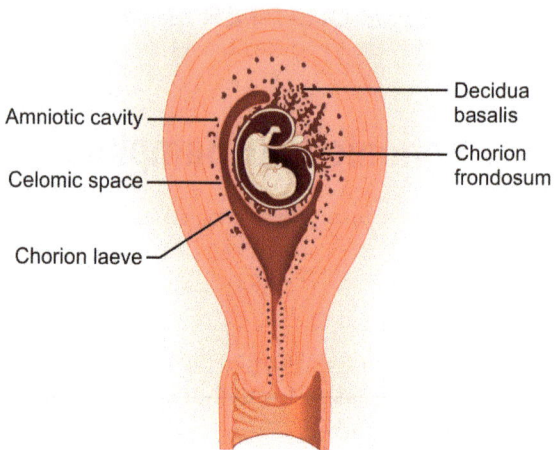

Fig. 9.1: Diagrammatic representation of the first trimester anatomy associated with chorionic villus sampling. At this gestational age the amnion and chorion have not yet fused and are separated by the extraembryonic celom. Beneath the developing chorion frondosum is the vascular decidua basalis.

If it is >3 mm there is increased risk of chromosomal abnormality specifically trisomy 21 and its presence should alert laboratory to perform rapid karyotyping by direct preparation
- On ultrasound chorion frondosum appears as hyperechoic homogeneous area and it should be accurately located prior to sampling (Figs. 9.2 and 9.3). Umbilical cord insertion can be determined for confirmation
- In the presence of uterine contraction the procedure should be delayed as it alters the shape of uterus and pulls the placental site to unusual location
- The bladder should be sufficiently full to allow adequate visualization but overfilling makes procedure difficult.

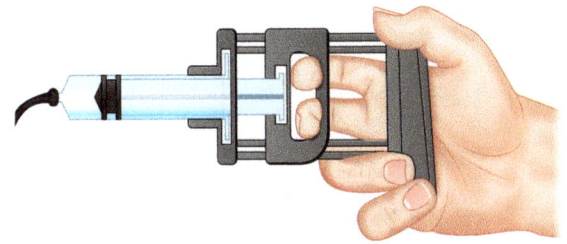

Fig. 9.2: Diagrammatic representation of hand grip used by some operators to facilitate transabdominal sampling.

SAMPLING DEVICES

Transcervical Catheter

Most frequently used catheter has a polyethylene outer sheath with an internal diameter of 0.89 mm. A stainless steel stylet fits snugly through the catheter to add sufficient rigidity for adequate passage through the cervix and into the frondosum. The stylet has a blunt end that protrudes slightly beyond catheter and prevents sharp edges from potentially perforating the membrane. The catheter has a Ruer Rok end so that syringe can be applied at the time of sampling.

A 20 mL syringe is used to apply suction once the catheter is in place; 5 mL of tissue with heparin should be aspirated into the syringe so that villi can be retrieved directly into this transport medium. The heparin prevents clotting of small amount of blood that is unavoidably retrieved.

Transabdominal Needle

- *Single needle*: 2.20 gauge spinal needle, 9 cm needle is sufficient, for obese patient 13 cm or 15 cm

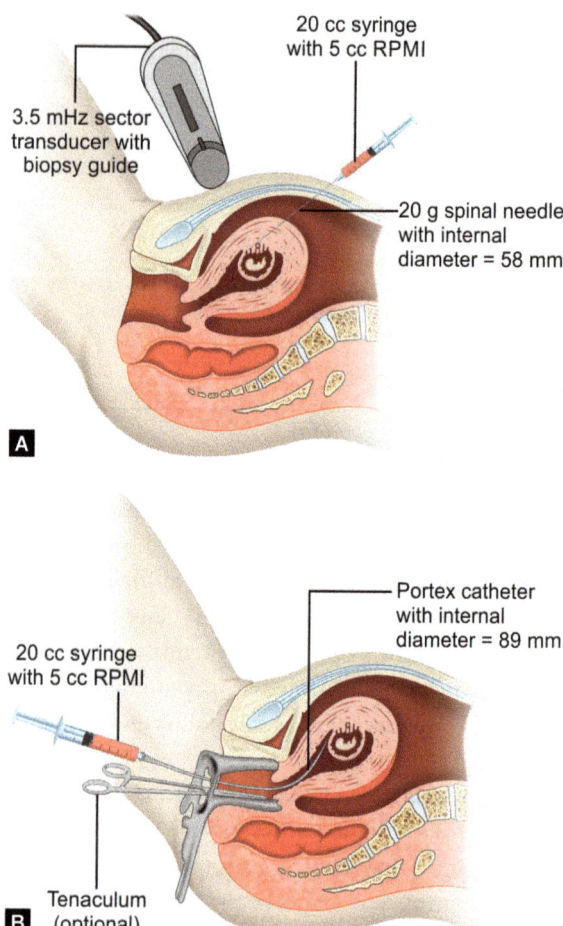

Figs. 9.3A and B: Diagrammatic representations of (A) transabdominal and (B) transcervical chorionic villus sampling.

- *Double needles*
  - Outer guide needle 18 gauge thin wall needle or 16–17 gauge standard needle
  - Sampling needle is same as in single needle technique.

Sampling Techniques

Both transcervical and transabdominal technique require 2 persons.

One individual performing the sampling and other doing the ultrasound guidance.

Transcervical Sampling

- Patient is placed in lithotomy position
- Vaginal area is prepared with povidone iodine solution
- Sims' speculum is entered and cervix directly wiped with antiseptic
- Anterior lip of cervix is held
- A gentle bend is made in the distal 3–5 cm of the catheter to accommodate insertion through cervical os and into frondosum
- The catheter is inserted till internal os is reached (slight loss in resistance)
- Allow the sonographer to image the tip
- The tip should be pointed in the correct direction. An interior position can be approached by pulling speculum downward which will move the catheter tip upward and into the proper location
- Once the tip is in the place, the catheter is gently advanced into the chorion frondosum under direct visualization the catheter should continue to be placed parallel to the chorionic plate through full length of the frondosum

- Once in place, the stylet is removed, medium filled syringe is attached and around 10-20 mL of pressure is applied
- The chorionic villi can be easily identified in the syringe by holding it up to light. They are seen as free floating, white tissue with fluffy branches (decidua is amorphous and has no branches)
- Maximum 2 attempts should be made.

Transabdominal Sampling

Single Needle Technique

- Abdomen is painted with povidone iodine
- Then the sampling path should be chosen such that the needle lies parallel to the chorion frondosum and will avoid any intervening bowel. The needle is inserted through abdominal wall into the myometrium
- Once the needle is within the myometrium the angle is readjusted so that the tip is parallel to chorion plate and pass through majority of the frondosum
- Once within the placenta the stylet is removed and a medium filled syringe is attached
- Villi are aspirated.

Double Needle Technique

- The abdomen is painted with povidone iodine. The anticipated path is also same as in single needle
- The outer gauge needle is inserted through the myometrium up to the edge of chorion frondosum
- Stylet is removed and sampling needle is inserted through guide needle into chorion frondosum
- Syringe with medium and continuous suction is applied.

Choosing Appropriate Technique

Both are equally safe. The best approach is the one in which the catheter or needle can be inserted parallel to chorion frondosum with the smallest amount of uterine or placental manipulation.

In General

Transcervical is painless. It is better for anteverted or midposition uterus with posterior placenta or retroverted uterus with anterior placenta

Cervical polyp or any cervical pathology is contraindication to transcervical approach.

Transabdominal approach is suited for anteverted uterus with inferior or fundal placenta.

In case of retroverted uterus with posterior placenta. Both transcervical or transabdominal are difficult. In these either transvesical or through anterior fornix or by manual anteriorization of uterus.

CVS Sampling in Twin

- Sample near cord insertion
- Combine transcervical and transabdominal approach to avoid confirmation of one sample of villi from coexisting fetus.

Complication

- Pregnancy loss
- Bleeding
- Rupture of membrane
- Infection
- Preterm labor

- Abruptio placentae
- IUGR.

How to Avoid Complication

- Decrease number of attempts
- Do not attempt in presence of uterine contraction
- Proper infection prevention techniques.

10
CHAPTER

Amniocentesis

INTRODUCTION

Amniocentesis was introduced in clinical practice in 19th century for treatment of polyhydramnios subsequently, it was used for amniography. Later in 1950's it was used as parental diagnostic test.

Real time ultrasonography added refinement and safety to the procedure allowing continuous monitoring of the needle position inside the amniotic cavity. The relative simplicity of the method and wide spread availability of ultrasonographic equipment and expertise made amniocentesis the most widely used invasive method of prenatal diagnosis.

INDICATIONS

Purpose	Indication
Late first and second trimester diagnosis	a. Cytogenetic diagnosis b. Diagnosis of neural tube defects c. Diagnosis of metabolic disorders
Last second and third trimester diagnosis	a. Evaluation of severity of isoimmunization b. Evaluation of fetal lung maturity c. Diagnosis of intraamniotic infection d. Confirmation of ruptured membrane
Therapeutic	a. Drainage of polyhydramnios b. Medical treatment of fetal disorder

Amniocentesis for Cytogenetic Diagnosis

Indication

- Women 35 years of age and older
- Couples with chromosomal rearrangement
- Previous offspring affected by chromosomal disorder
- Women carrying X-linked disease
- Parents with a recessive gene for metabolic disease or hemoglobinopathy.

Time

After 15 weeks commonly 16 and 18 weeks.

MIDTRIMESTER AMNIOCENTESIS TECHNIQUE

Selecting Puncture Site

USG is performed before to:
- Determine number of fetuses
- Viability of fetus
- Placental location
- Amount of amniotic fluid
- Presence of uterine or fetal anomalies

A site of puncture avoiding placental tissue or umbilical cord in the needle path is selected transplacental puncture are associated with an increased risk of pregnancy loss and maternal cell contamination.

In case transplacental puncture is necessary, the place with the least amount of placental tissue should be selected.

Selecting a Needle

- Depends on size of the patient and the amount of fluid to be retrieved
- 20–22 gauge spinal needle with standard length 8.89 cm including the heels.

Special Points

- Obese patients require longer needle
- Small bore needle prolong time
- Large bore needle increases fetal loss
- Needles with side orifice increase flow rate to double.

Monitoring the Needle Insertion and Placement

- After selecting puncture site asepsis of skin is performed with wide boundaries and field is draped
- Two approaches

USG guided	USG monitored
Preselection of puncture site with ultrasound before blind insertion of needle	Continuous monitoring of needle insertion and fetal movement with real time ultrasound. This reduces bloody and dry taps

Transducers

Non-staining coupling gel is applied to the transducer surface before placing it inside a sterile glove or plastic bag. A sterile coupling agent is then applied to patient's skin and the puncture site is re-evaluated.

Selection of Transducers

Convex or Sector	Linear array
1. Allows visualization of entire needle all the way from patients skin to amniotic cavity	Gloved finger is placed at the puncture site directly under the transducer
2. Puncture site will be located in front and a few cm away from the transducer	
3. Needle must enter at an angle to reach amniotic fluid pocket underneath transducer	

Amniotic Fluid Aspiration

- Once the stylet is removed an extension tube (which allows the needle to float free in the amniotic cavity, decreasing chance of fetal injury) is attached to the heels of the needle and connected to the syringe
- First 0.5 mL of amniotic fluid is discarded to avoid maternal contamination
- After aspiration stylet is relocated needle is removed
- Fetal cardiac activity is documented.

Early Amniocentesis

It is performed before 15 weeks of gestation. This allows the diagnosis of anomalies at a time when suction termination is still possible and before fetal movements are perceived.

It gives opportunity to screen for neural tube defects, by measurement of AFP and acetyl cholinesterase after 13 weeks and there is no need for major operative changes contrary to CVS.

Early amniocentesis can be done at 7 weeks but abortion rate will be more than as compared to 13 weeks. Largest number of viable cells are present between 13 to 16 weeks.

Modification in Technique

- Small-bore spinal needle is used
- Recommended fluid to be withdrawn 1 mL per week of gestation
- First 0.5–1 mL of fluid is discarded to prevent maternal contamination or first 2 mL can be sent for AFP or acetyl choline sterase
- Transvaginal approach provides high resolution and easy access to amniotic sac, but has more risk of bacterial and fungal contamination

- *Amniofilteration*: It has been proposed as a means to retrieve amniotic fluid cells in early amniocentesis is without removing a relatedly large proportion of amniotic fluid. A filter paper with appropriate pore size is interposed between syringe and needle, the amniotic fluid is recirculated back into amniotic cavity and cells are retrieved from filter membrane.

Complication

- Fetal loss
- Fetal injury
- Amniotic fluid leakage
- Bloody taps
- Fetomaternal transfusion.

Amniocentesis and Isoimmunization

Fetal red blood cells contain D antigen on their surface and are capable of immunizing Rh negative mother after a fetomaternal transfusion in the mid trimester. WHO and ACOG have recommended the administrates of anti-D IgG after mid trimester. Dose by WHO 50 µg, ACOG 300 mg. Efficacy and long term safety is not proven.

Amniocentesis in Multiple Gestation

- More incidence of fetal chromosomal anomalies and neural tube defects have been found in twin gestation than in singleton pregnancy
- Possible outcome risk and management alternatives need to be discussed with patient
- If only one fetus is affected the option available include abortion of both fetus, continuation of pregnancy or selective feticide of affected fetus

- An important step is the topographic motion of the fetus. This becomes important where discrepant results are reported and selective feticide is considered. Identification of fetus should be based on their relationship to maternal pelvis
- After amniotic fluid is obtained from the first sac and before removing the needle dye is injected into the cavity
- Indigo carmine is dye of choice. The use of methylene blue is discouraged because of risk of fetal hemolytic anemia due to methemoglobinemia and possible association with gastrointestinal obstruction. Clear amniotic fluid should be obtained when second sac is punctured
- Single needle insertion can be done in twin amniocentesis. The puncture site clear of placental tissue demonstrating both gestational sacs and the intra-amniotic membrane is selected with real time ultrasound
- The most proximal sac is aspirated first; the stylet is replaced into the needle and advanced under ultrasound guidance through the intra-amniotic membrane into second sac finally, fluid is aspirated from second sac
- Two needle aspiration may be performed simultaneously by two operators into two separate sacs under direct ultrasonographic guidance.

Difficulties

- One sac behind the other
- Amniotic membrane cannot be identified.

Amniocentesis for Diagnosis of Microbial Invasion of Amniotic Cavity

Amniotic cavity is normally sterile and isolation of any microorganism from the amniotic fluid consists evidence of microbial invasion.

Microbial invasion of amniotic cavity (MIAC) can insist even in the absence of clinical signs and symptoms of injection and has been implicated as a causative phenomenon for both preterm labor with intact membrane and premature rupture of membrane. Early identification of MIAC is important since neonates born to mothers with intra-amniotic injection are at higher risk for injection complication. The diagnosis of MIAC relies upon examination of amniotic fluid.

Techniques

- Transabdominal amniocentesis
- Transcervical retrieval either by needle puncturing of membrane or aspiration through intrauterine catheter.

Transcervical is associated with risk of contamination with vaginal flora, and is contraindicated in patients with preterm labour and patients with PROMs not in labour.

Diagnosis

Amniotic fluid culture (gold standard): Amniotic fluid should be transported to laboratory in capped syringe. This maximizes the recovery of anaerobic bacteria.

Rapid Diagnosis of Intra-amniotic Injection

- Amniotic fluid gram stain (most rapid)
- Amniotic fluid WBC count
- Glucose concentration in the amniotic fluid
- Amniotic fluid microphage derived cytokines.

CHAPTER 11

Multifetal Reduction

INTRODUCTION

Over the past 25-30 years starting with ovulation induction and ever evolving ART practices like IUI, IVF, ICSI the number of multifetal pregnancy is increasing (Fig. 11.1). This increase in multifetal pregnancy has been from 1.25% in spontaneous pregnancies to 5-8% with clomiphene induced cycles and is nearly 30% in patients using exogenous gonadotropins for superovulation for subfertility.

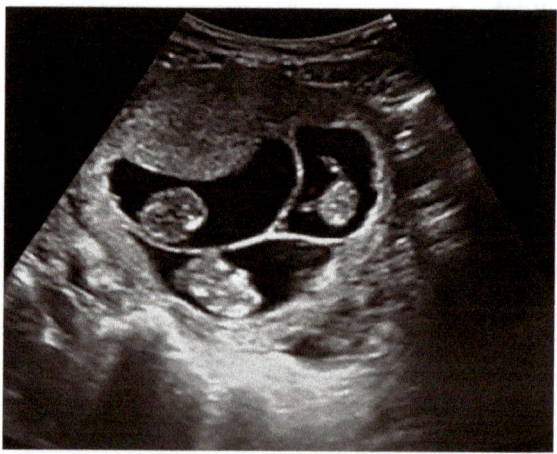

Fig. 11.1: Ultrasound picture of triplet pregnancy.

Multifetal Reduction

Though with lot of debate internationally, rationale has come up for ovulation induction (OI), IUI and number of embryos transfer in IVF cycles with even going up to single embryo transfer but still multiple pregnancy is a inevitable situation even in today's scenarios.

Multiple pregnancy is not all good situation for the infertile couples who conceive with difficulty because of risks associated with high order pregnancy like premature labor, early pregnancy loses, diabetes, hypertensive disorders, placental abruption, placenta previa and for fetus early miscarriage or late miscarriage most commonly, low birth weight, IUGR. Preterm births, IUGR leading to prolong stay in NICU increasing the financial burden on parents (Fig. 11.2).

To reduce this, high order pregnancies are dealt now-a-days by high-risk pregnancy units by multifetal reduction or embryo reduction. It needs a lot of counseling and emotional support of couples who might have conceived after a long period of infertility.

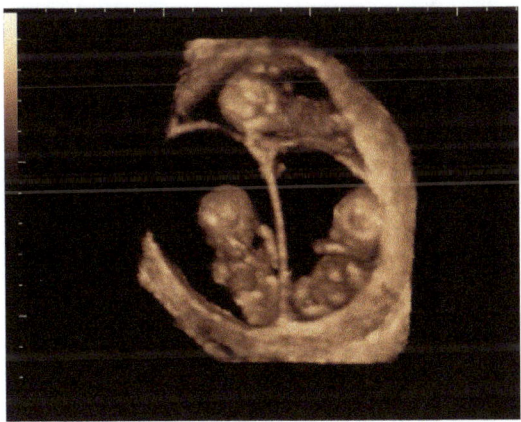

Fig. 11.2: 3D image of triplets.

In 2006, International Federation of Gynecologists and Obstetricians (FIGO) Committee Report stated that "multiple pregnancies of an order of magnitude higher than twins involves great danger for the woman's health and also for her fetuses, which are likely to be delivered prematurely with a high risk of either dying or suffering damage," and that "where such pregnancies arise, it may be considered ethically preferable to reduce the number of fetuses rather than to do nothing".

EMBRYO REDUCTION—THE PROCEDURE

Embryo reduction is performed after describing all risks associated like early abortion in IV sedation or GA under propofol with one day stay. Routes used are transabdominal, transcervical, transvaginal (Figs. 11.3 and 11.4). Transabdominal is done at early first or second trimester at 11–13 weeks with a

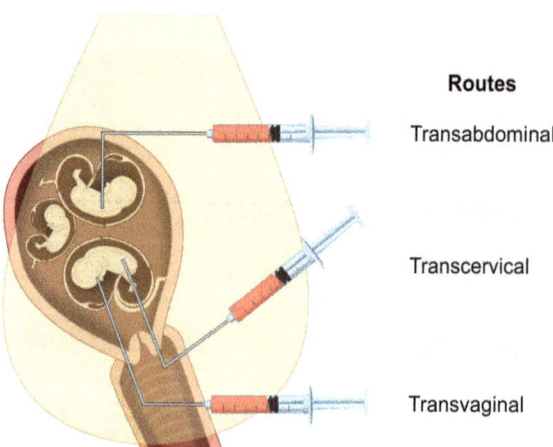

Fig. 11.3: Routes of fetal reduction.

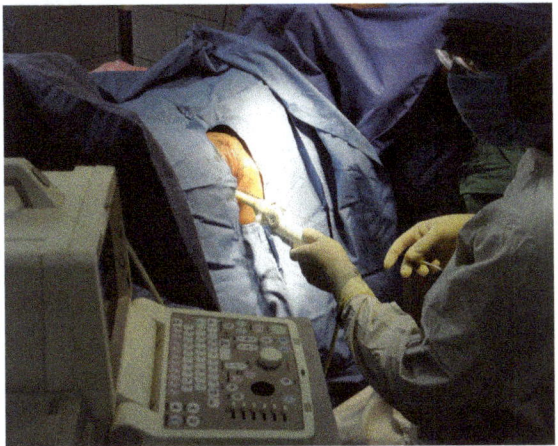

Fig. 11.4: Procedure of fetal reduction.

transthoracic injection of cardiotoxic drug into selected fetus. Transcervical aspiration of the gestational sac is done, it may be associated with an increased incidence of abortions due to infection introduced from the cervix or cervical incompetence brought about by cervical dilatation and is therefore not recommended.

Transvaginal is more convenient to perform and more so can be done at early gestation < 11 weeks and now-a-days we are even advocating and performing between 6–8 weeks.

The most accessible gestational sac is chosen, and the fetal heart is visualized and aligned with the puncture guideline on the screen. For early reductions 6–8 weeks an oocyte retrieval needle, is advanced sharply toward the fetal heart (Fig. 11.5).

At > 9 weeks 0.5–3 mL of KCl (15%) is injected. In most cases, the fetal echoes disappear completely and the sac remains of the same size or slightly smaller, but empty of fetal parts.

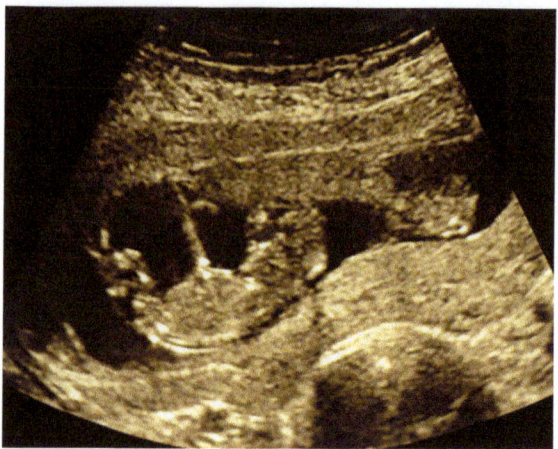

Fig. 11.5: Needle in the fetus.

After making sure that there are no more pulsations, we withdraw the needle.

Follow-up scan of the patient is done after 24 hours and then after 1 week.

Which method to choose? At what gestation? Pros and cons.
While choosing a method most important is convenience and expertise of the operating person.

Its Kovitz et al. in 1992 who described two cases of multifetal reduction without the use of an embryotoxic substance. First, they applied suction only to stop fetal pulsations and not to aspirate the embryonic tissues. Second, they partially aspirated the amniotic fluid. They concluded it to be a better method than with embryotoxic substance.

The rate of miscarriage in Mansour study using the modified technique was 8.8% in Cairo in Egyptian IVF center. This was less than the 12.6% loss rate reported by Sebire et al. in their series of 127 multifetal pregnancies undergoing embryo reduction and also less than the 13.7% loss rate reported by Evans et al. in a multicenter study of multifetal embryo reductions.

A study by Lee on 148 patients also concluded that as per them, they called non KCl early group faired better. The study was a retrospective comparative study of different modalities comprised of two components of the MFPR procedure, i.e., the use of an embryotoxic agent, and the timing of procedure.

KCl as an embryotoxic substance has a high fetal wastage rate (30%). One explanation for the lower miscarriage rate using the modified technique is that we performed it after gaining more experience and at an earlier gestational age. It has been reported that it is feasible to complete the procedure as early as 6 weeks' gestation, although it might be preferable to wait until 8 weeks or later for fear of the natural phenomenon known as "vanishing twin." The advocates like us for early reduction say that performing the procedure as early as possible without excessive concern about the phenomenon of vanishing twins because two gestational sacs will remain. Even if one sac vanishes, a singleton pregnancy will result.

Another factor that plays a role in reducing the miscarriage rate using the modified technique is that most of the embryonic tissue is aspirated at an early gestation age. Aspiration leaves a minimal amount of necrotic tissue, which may have detrimental effects on the remaining gestational sacs. In the beginning, it was difficult to imagine that it was possible to aspirate an embryo of 6–8 weeks with visible pulsations. However, the embryo at this stage is composed of three primary germ layers (ectoderm, endoderm, and mesoderm) folding to form the head, tail, and lateral body folds, and these soft tissues and membranes are easily removed with repeated suction.

One of the causes of pregnancy loss in reduced twins is the development of an inflammatory response to the resorbing necrotic fetoplacental tissues, with the resulting release of cytokines and prostaglandins. High concentrations of α-fetoprotein (AFP) are found in the amniotic fluid of twin pregnancies after spontaneous death of one of the fetuses, as reported by Bass et al. and in reduced twins.

Another reason for the lower miscarriage rate is that the injection of KCl is not strictly limited to the fetal heart. During injection, the fetus is sometimes pushed away from the needle and KCl diffuses into the amniotic sac; consequently it may diffuse to the adjacent gestational sacs. Toxic effects of KCl on the remaining fetuses have been reported by Tabsh et al. and Wapner et al.

In comparison with the nonreduced twins, the outcome of the twins resulting from the modified reduction technique was not significantly different with regard to the miscarriage rate, fetal wastage rate, mean gestational age, and birth weight. In 1996, Smith-Levitin et al. demonstrated that reduced twins were similar to nonreduced twins conceived with assisted reproduction in all variables studied.

It was also noted in this series that the early (<12 weeks) miscarriage rate was only 2.6%, which is similar to that of early amniocentesis in singleton pregnancies (2.2%). This leads to the assumption that most miscarriages associated with multifetal reduction are not the consequence of spontaneous loss, nor are they directly due to the procedure and the use of needles in the reduction.

The mean gestational age at delivery (36.9 ± 2.45 weeks) of the twins resulting from the modified technique was similar to that of the nonreduced twins conceived by assisted reproduction (36.5 ± 2.58 weeks). This finding is probably due to the minimal amount of necrotic tissues remaining after reduction and thus the smaller likelihood that their resorption could trigger labor.

J Haas very recently in his study in 2015 again gave same insight but gave a different conclusion. In MPR from triplets, an apparent benefit was observed for early MPR in preterm deliveries before 37 weeks, whereas, in MPR from high-order pregnancies, a benefit was observed for late MPR in deliveries before 32 weeks. Perinatal outcomes of twin pregnancies after early and late MPR seem to be grossly similar. They said optimal timing for multifetal reduction depends on other factors, namely, the selectivity of the procedure and patient's preference.

Another question in multiple pregnancy is to reduce to twin or singleton. Our Indian patients always prefer reduction to twin only but sometimes for medical condition one has to reduce to single also.

In our study between 2010–2014, MFR at our center (Rainbow Hospital, Agra) was done of 148 cases from which 9 were quadruplets to twins, 124 of triplet to twins and remaining twins to singleton of 4 cases. Loss was noted in 25% cases of singleton pregnancies although rate of preterm labor were almost same in all three groups.

	Number (n)	Outcome immediate loss	Late loss	Preterm delivery	Term delivery
No. of MFPR	148				
No. of quads to twins	09	01(11.1%)		02(22.2%)	06(66.6%)
No. of triplets to twins	135	17(12.5%)	12(8%)	27(28.1%)	67(69.7%)
No. of twins to singletons	04	01(25%)		01(25%)	02(50%)

CONCLUSION

So now we all accept that embryo reduction is part of ever expanding infertility practice. One needs to get expertise and choose the best method in which one is confident and definitely early reduction is best mode both for mother and fetus as well as obstetricians to manage.

12
CHAPTER

Prenatal Diagnosis and Therapeutic Techniques in Twin Pregnancies

In case of twins there is evidence that fluid must be obtained separately from each sac and investigated for any anomaly.

DIAGNOSIS OF CHORIONICITY

Before 8 weeks, monozygotic twins will appear in the same gestational sac and intertwin membrane is difficult to visualize.

From 9 to 12 weeks, dichorionic twins will be separated by a thick membrane, whose insertion of the placenta/uterine wall will have a characteristic 'Y' shape. Mono-chorionic twins will be separated by a thin hairy membrane inserting sharply on the placenta.

After 15 weeks, differentiating mono and dichorionic twins becomes less accurate. Different genders, separate placental masses and thickness of the membranes may not be the sufficient criteria.

The most appropriate method are the DNA techniques by fetal tissue especially before gender is apparent.

AMNIOCENTESIS

Traditionally, amniocentesis in a twin pregnancy involved puncture of the first sac, withdrawal of amniotic fluid, injection of a dye and then a new needle insertion to puncture the second sac. The disadvantage of this method is that, two skin and uterine entries are required, increasing the potential for complications and secondly, methylene blue dye injection may cause neonatal bowel occlusions.

In order to avoid the second puncture, which could enhance uterine activity and increase the risk of intra-amniotic infection, we recommend the *single needle insertion technique.*

- The site of needle insertion is determined by the position of the membrane separating the two sacs
- After entry into the first sac and aspiration of the amniotic fluid, the needle is advanced through the dividing membrane into the second sac
- To avoid contamination of the first sac fluid, the first 1 mL of the fluid from the first sac is discarded with needle still in the second sac
- This method is simple, less traumatic and with fewer complications than the traditional method.

CHORIONIC VILLUS SAMPLING

A combination of ultrasound, fetal sex determination and genetic studies using polymorphic markers may be required to differentiate the two samples, however a single sample is performed when the twins are monochorionic.

Chorionic villus sampling is preferably performed at 9–12 weeks chorionicity is easily determined at this stage and for dichorionicity, two separate samples from each placenta is preferred.

When chorionicity is uncertain, sampling at the insertion of the umbilical cord can be helpful, although it could theoretically increase the risk of fetal loss.

At the time of the procedure, a detailed transabdominal ultrasound evaluation is done delineating:
- Crown rump length of each fetus
- Location of each placenta
- Margins of each placenta relative to any gestational sac
- Location and thickness of the dividing membrane
- Sampling method—single or double is determined.

Fetal Blood Sampling

This is facilitated by precise cord localization and therefore facilitates identification of a malformed/chromosomally abnormal fetus. Blood subgroup determination in each sample is a useful adjacent to the rapid diagnosis of zygosity.

Twin to Twin Transfusion Syndrome

Ultrasound examination demonstrates monochorionic diamniotic twin pregnancies with discordant fetal sizes.

The larger twin (recipient) has a distended bladder with polyhydramnios, whereas the smaller twin (donor) has an empty bladder with anhydramnios and fetus appears fixed to the placenta or uterine wall.

The fetal BPD/HC/AC/FL are measured and fetal weight calculated. The intertwin difference in weight is expressed as a percentage of the weight of the recipient. The degree of polyhydramnios is assessed by measuring the deepest vertical pool.

Amniodrainage

In case of polyhydramnios an 18 gauge needle is introduced into the uterus under ultrasound guidance and the amniotic fluid is allowed to drain into a sterile bag through a plastic tube attached to the hub of the needle over 40-120 min until there is subjective normalization of amniotic fluid volume on ultrasound examination.

Patients are assessed every week and further amniodrainage is performed if there is recurrence of polyhydramnios.

LASER COAGULATION OF PLACENTAL ANASTOMOSIS

A detailed ultrasound with color flow mapping is first performed.

This will localize the placenta, the inter-twin amniotic membrane, umbilical cord insertion site and the communicating blood vessels on the chorionic plate.

The appropriate site of maternal abdomen is chosen such that it avoids injury to the placenta or fetuses and allows access to the suspected area of vascular communications.

Under continuous ultrasound visualization, a rigid 2 mm diameter fetoscope with cannula is introduced into the amniotic cavity of the recipient twin. A 400 µm diameter ND YAG laser is introduced down the side arm of the cannula, 1 cm beyond the tip of fetoscope and the crossing vessels are coagulated by administration of total of 1000-4500 J delivered by 3-5 shots using output of 30-50 W at a distance of 1 cm.

Subsequently, amniotic fluid is drained to normalize its volume.

Acardiac Twin: Selective Feticide in Monochorionic Pregnancies

Acardiac twin is the extreme manifestation of twin to twin transfusion syndrome and is found in approximately 1% of monozygotic twin pregnancies.

This twin disorder is called twin - reversed arterial perfusion (TRAP) sequence. There is disruption of the normal vascular perfusion and development of the recipient twin due to umbilical artery to artery anastomosis with the donor twin.

At least 50% of donor twins die due to CCF or severe preterm delivery (polyhydramnios) or because of associated multiple anomalies.

Prenatal treatment by aminodrainage or administration of indomethacin to the mother, prevents only polyhydramnios.

Attempts to reduce incidence of CCF/Intrauterine or neonatal deaths are by surgical removal of acardiac twin or occlusion of umbilical cord. Selective removal of acardiac twin by hysteroscopy was not successful.

To arrest umbilical blood flow a number of procedures were done like ultrasound guided injection thrombogenic coils or fibrin, endoscopic laser coagulation which is feasible if the patient reports before 20 weeks of pregnancy.

Embolization of both the arterial and venous system can be achieved by ultrasound guided cordocentesis using different approaches and materials.

Endoscopic cord ligation involves the use of two ports (under GA) one for endoscope and one for introduction of suture.

The suture is passed around the cord and tied extra corporeally.

Though, there is risk of neonatal death due to premature labor or premature rupture of membranes.

CHAPTER 13

Gynecology Procedures

INTRODUCTION (FIGS. 13.1 AND 13.2)

A p/s and p/v is still the mainstay of any gynecological examination, however the results are subjective, addition of TVS has given an objective component and is a marriage of palpation and imaging, addition of color gives physiological

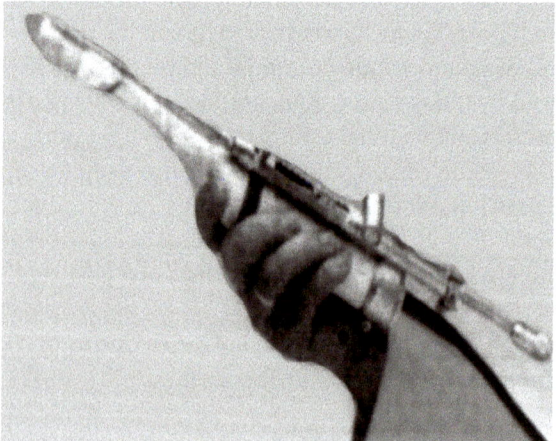

Fig. 13.1: Transvaginal probe with biopsy guide and needle.

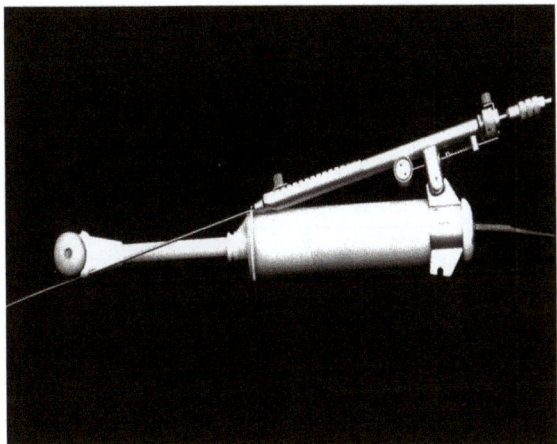

Fig. 13.2: Transvaginal probe with biopsy guide and needle.

information and 3D has added a new dimension to examining the pelvis, however, all these are anatomical and physiological diagnosis and to get a histopathological diagnosis, the needle has to be introduced in the target organ to obtain a sample for HPE–Interventional gynecological sonography.

- Counseling
- Written consent
- Minor OT set-up
- Anesthesia
- Proper needles
- Biopsy guide
- Prophylactic antibiotics
- Pre-and post-procedure TVS and color Doppler scan.

ADNEXAL CYSTIC MASSES (FIGS. 13.3 TO 13.10)

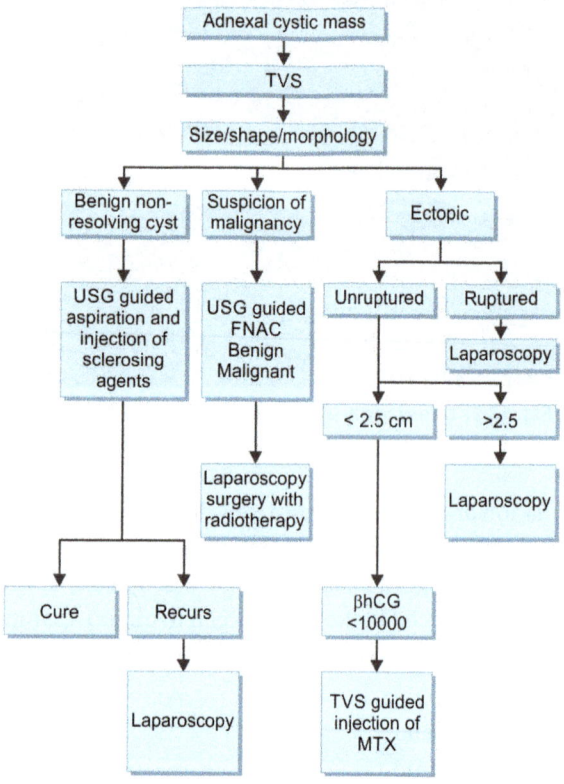

Indications for ultrasound guided puncture of adnexal cysts.
- Is it necessary?
- Is it possible?
- Is it acceptable?
- Is it enough?

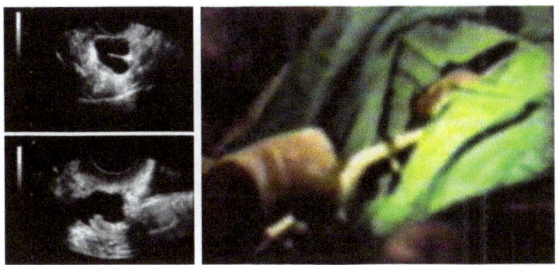

Fig. 13.3: Drainage of a hydrosalpinx.

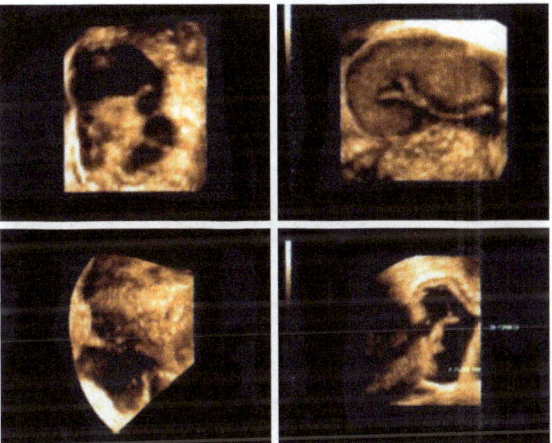

Fig. 13.4: 3D ultrasound evaluation of the tube (Hydro and pyosalpinx).

Technique

- Counseling
- Written consent
- USG evaluation

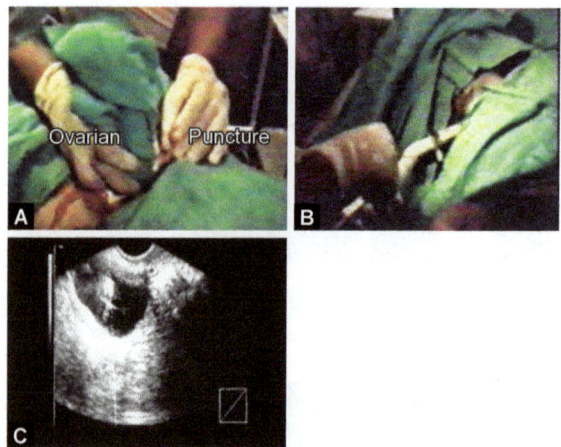

Figs. 13.5A to C: Cyst puncture under ultrasound guidance.

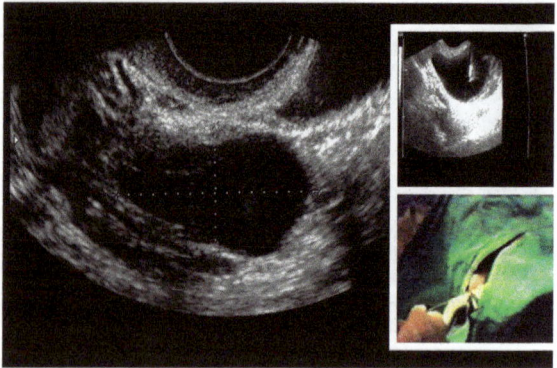

Fig. 13.6: Cyst puncture under ultrasound guidance.

- Minor OT procedure
- Anesthesia
- TAS or TVS

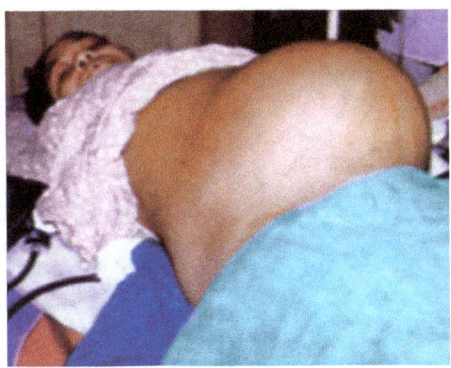

Fig. 13.7: Ovarian cyst puncture with a 28-week pregnancy.

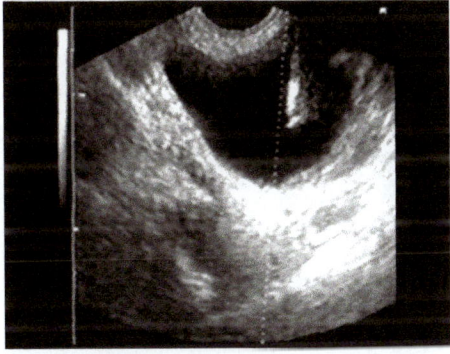

Fig. 13.8: Needle seen in ovarian cyst.

- Needles 17 to 20 gauge
- Aspiration pump
- Injection of sclerosing agents (Terramycin or ethoxysclerol)
- Cytological examination of cyst aspirated material
- Antibiotics
- Follow-up.

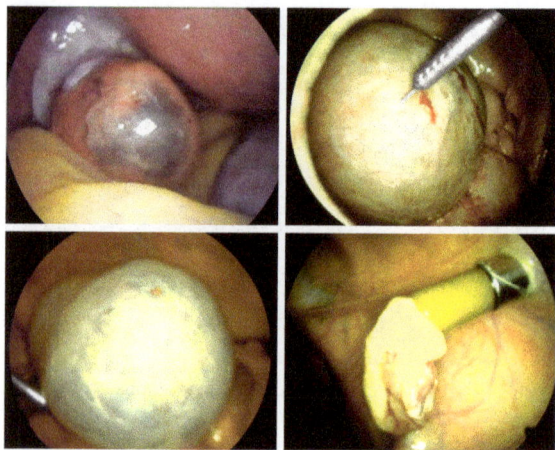

Fig. 13.9: Abnormal ovaries as seen on a laparoscope (laparoscopic ovarian cystectomy).

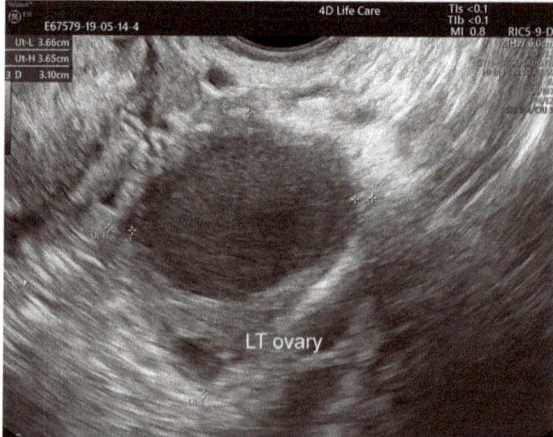

Fig. 13.10: Ovarian cyst with multiple coarse internal echoes (endometrioma) (Ground glass appearance).

PELVIC MASSES

Pelvic masses may arise from the genital tract or may be non-gynecological. They may be cystic, solid or mixed and may be infective or neoplastic.

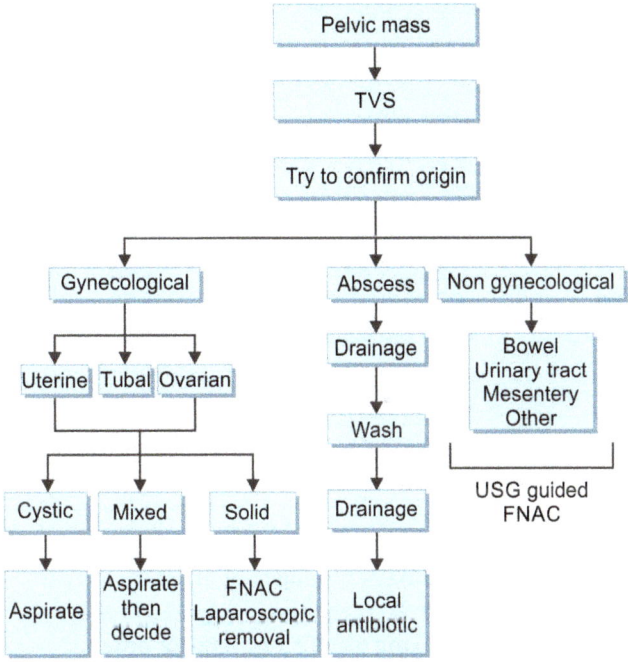

ECTOPIC PREGNANCY MANAGEMENT (FIGS. 13.11 TO 13.16)

There is today a non-surgical method for treating ectopic pregnancies which have not ruptured and where patients are hemodynamically stable.

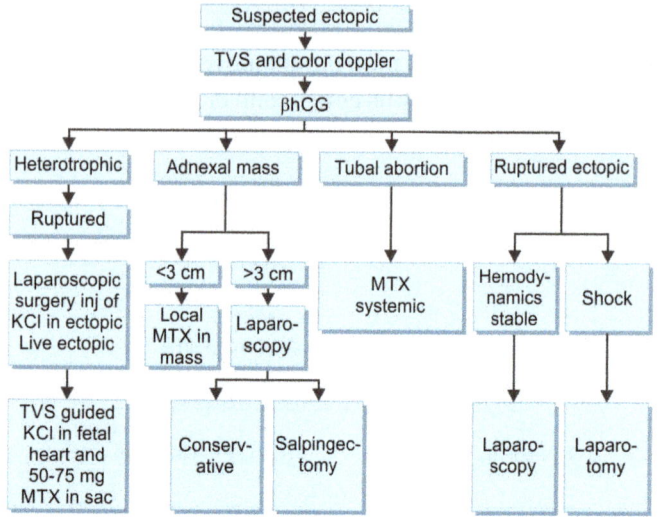

Technique

- Diagnosis
- Counseling
- Written consent
- Anesthesia
- TVS guided needle 17–20 gauge put in sac
- Salpingocentesis
- Injection of 50–75 mg of MTX or RU486 or others
- Prophylactic antibiotic
- Baseline blood tests and βhCG levels
- Monitoring treatment by serial TVS color Doppler and βhCG
- > 80% success
- > 70% spontaneous tube recanalization
- A very good, safe and effective treatment for early unruptured ectopic pregnancy.

Gynecology Procedures

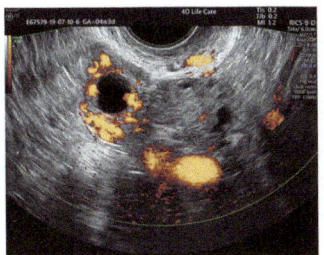

Fig. 13.11: Ectopic pregnancy

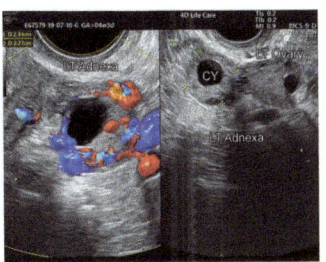

Fig. 13.12: Ring of fire sign

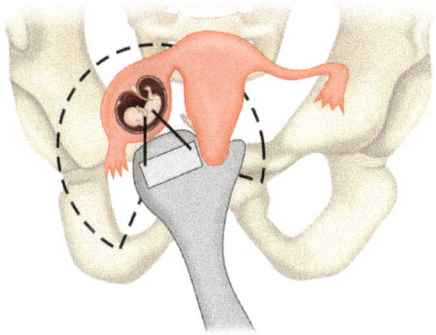

Fig. 13.13: Technique for management of an ectopic pregnancy.

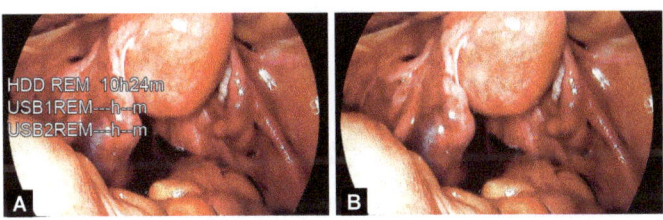

Figs. 13.14A and B: Laparoscopic management of an ectopic pregnancy.

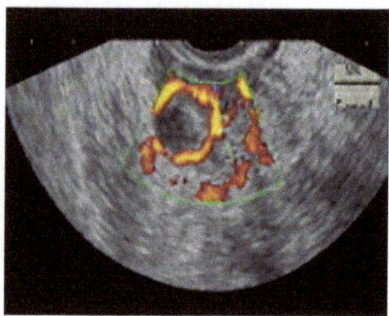

Fig. 13.15: Ectopic pregnancy as evaluated by a TVS and color Doppler.

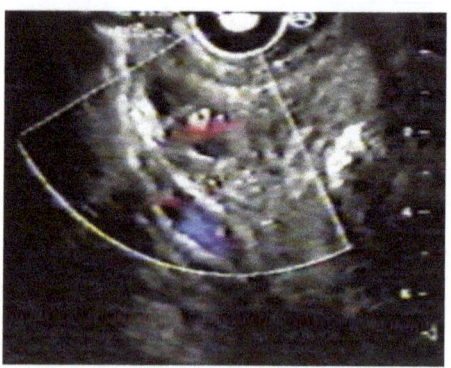

Fig. 13.16: Local injection in an ectopic pregnancy.

TRANSCERVICAL METROPLASTY (FIGS. 13.17 AND 13.18)

Congenital anomalies of the uterus are a major cause of recurrent pregnancy loss and even infertility.

A hysteroscopic correction of septa and lateral metroplasty is the gold standard treatment modality.

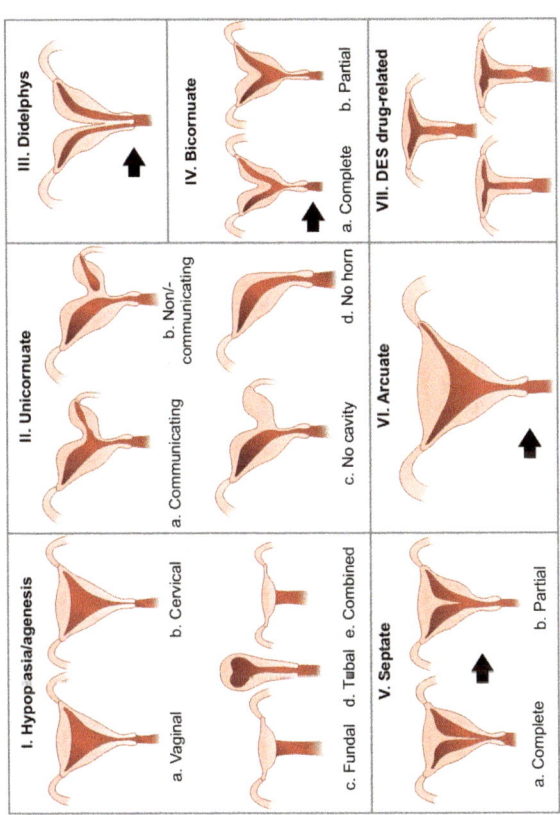

Fig. 13.17: ASRM classification.

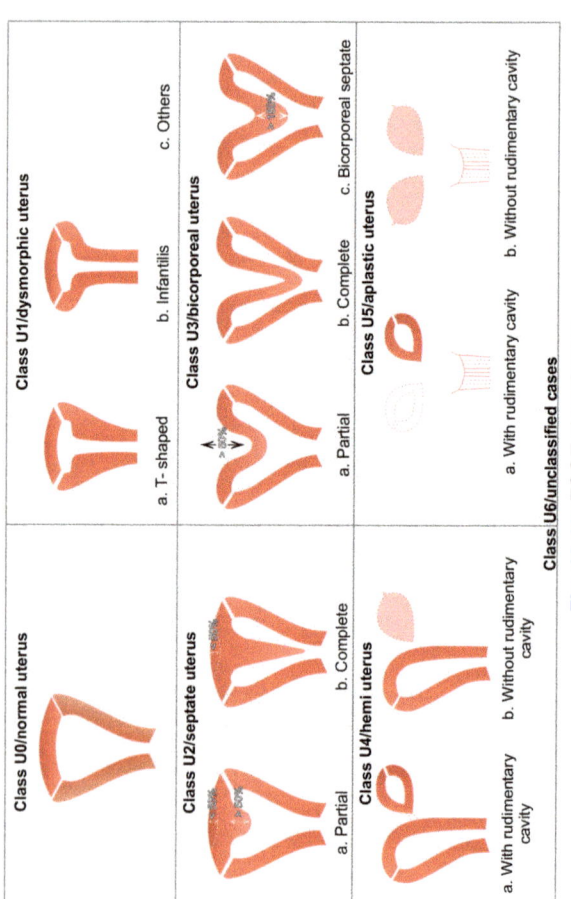

Fig. 13.18: ESGE classification.

The same treatment can be carried out under ultrasound guidance.

Improved resolution of machines have opened up new exciting possibility of septum resection as an OPD procedure under ultrasound guidance.

UROGYNECOLOGY (FIGS. 13.19 TO 13.21)

- Post-voiding residual volume
- Descent of bladder neck

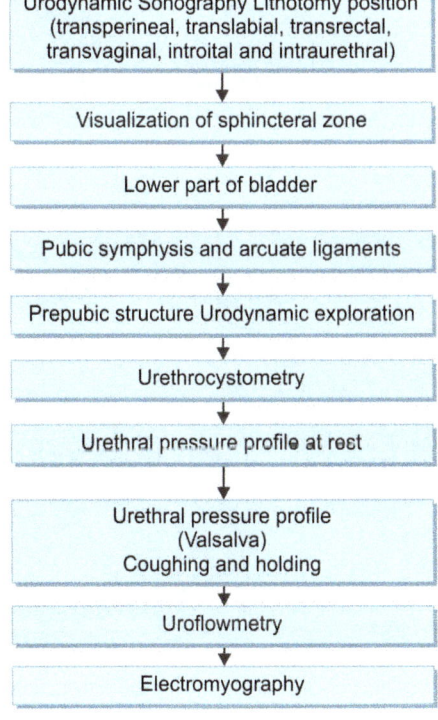

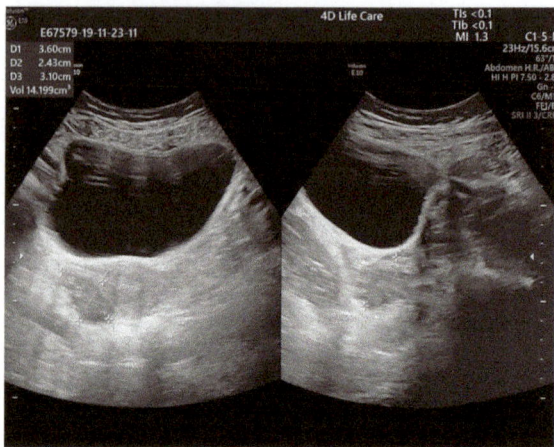

Fig. 13.19: Urinary bladder study in a normal female.

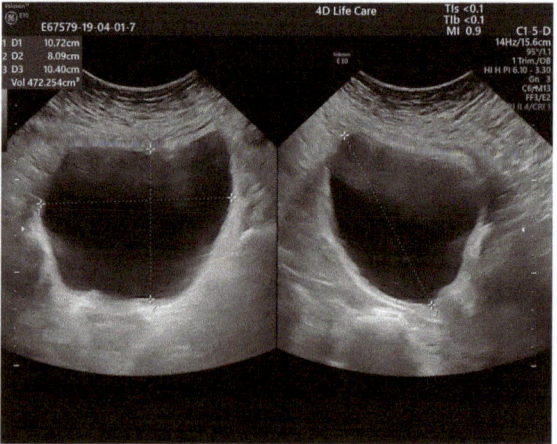

Fig. 13.20: Urinary bladder study in a female with incontinence (I).

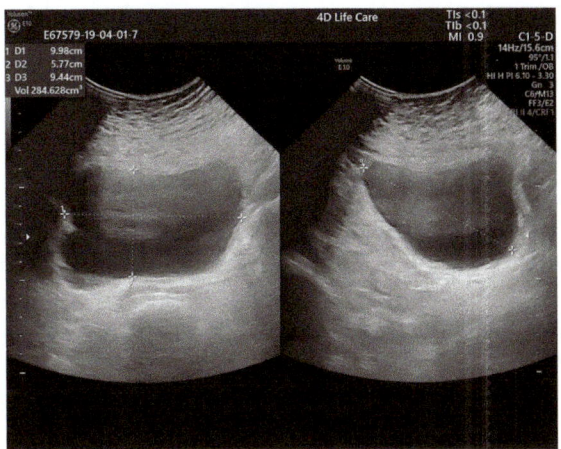

Fig. 13.21: Urinary bladder study in a female with incontinence (II).

Stress Incontinence Surgery and Ultrasound

Preoperative Assessment

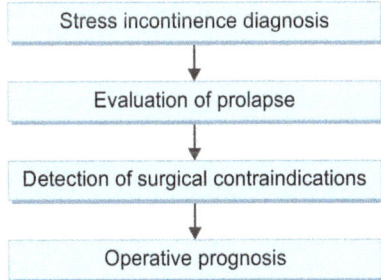

Peroperative

- Control of suspension position
- Tension of suspension

- Passage of instrument in Retzius space
- Urinary stress in continence evaluation
- Suprapubic vesical catheter.

Postoperative

- Anatomical modifications
- Visualization of exogenous tissues

Urodynamic ultrasound today can offer a reliable and safe and nonsatiation method to morphologically evaluate the female urinary tract.

14

CHAPTER

Ultrasound in Treatment of Adnexal Cystic Masses

Over the last few years there has been a shift of treatment of adnexal masses from laparotomy of adnexal masses to laparotomy to minimal invasive surgery.

ULTRASOUND GUIDED PUNCTURE OF ADNEXAL CYSTIC MASSES

Puncture of Benign Masses

Evidence-based medicine and experience suggests that puncture of benign ovarian neoplasms is not a satisfactory treatment as 30–40% of recurrences have been reported and some reporters have suggested that these may be precursors of ovarian cancer.

The indications of ultrasonographic management of adnexal masses can be summarized by asking 3 questions:
1. Is it necessary?
2. If necessary, is it possible and/or acceptable?
3. Is it enough?

Is any Surgical Approach Necessary?

It has been noted that if the adnexal mass is purely cystic it may be a functional cyst and they may spontaneous disappear without any surgical procedure.

Ultrasound puncture can be proposed as an alternative to expectant management of a 3 month treatment with oral contraceptive pills. There are several arguments against this.
- The classical delay of 3 months will be much too long in early ovarian cancer
- Follow up will be difficult especially in young patients
- It is similar for a patient to get her cyst aspirated and send for examination than, to comply with follow ups.

Is it Possible and/or Acceptable?

Preoperative selection is essential to make ultrasound guided puncture safe and acceptable.

Clinical Criteria

A detailed history is very useful in understanding the nature of the adnexal cyst.

It should include age, LMP, previous surgical history, history of PID, endometriosis or use of ovulation inducing drugs and diameter and bilaterally of the cyst.

Contraindications of USG Guided Puncture

- Patients more than 5 years after menopause except bilateral oophorectomy has been performed and a peritoneal cyst is suspected
- Patients whose ovarian activity is stopped by a medical treatment except those on GnRh analog treatment started two months ago.

Indications of USG Guided Puncture

- Patients where ovarian activity is not inhibited by any treatment
- Pregnant patients before 14 weeks of pregnancy

- Patients diagnosed previously with extensive pelvic adhesions and/or peritoneal cysts
- Postmenopausal women with adnexal cysts similar to those observed by the patient when she was menstruating regularly
- Very old patients in poor general condition.

Ultrasound Criteria

An USG guided puncture is generally proposed in entirely cystic masses and ultrasonographic appearance is related to pathological diagnosis. The factors favoring USG guided punctures are the following:
- The incidence of malignant tumor is low among entirely cystic adnexal masses
- With better resolution USG machines, some false negatives will be encountered
- The surgical diagnosis is still essential
- A USG guided puncture should be considered as an surgical procedure and be performed in the operation theater.

Conflicting attitudes have been reported in the ultrasonographic management of septated masses.
- A puncture is acceptable when diagnosis of functional cyst is likely especially in patients with ovarian hyperstimulation or patients with previous surgical history which suggests severe pelvic adhesions
- Some workers have included complex masses with thin septae
- USG puncture is contraindicated in masses with thick, septae or more complex appearances especially if there is evidence of neovascularization on color Doppler
- A preoperative CA 125 value may help in taking a decision.

Is it Enough?

Laparoscopic and ultrasonographic studies have shown a high recurrence rate (41-61%) after puncture of benign ovarian neoplasms. This rate is related to the cyst diameter and incomplete aspiration.

The appearance of fluid aspirated may lead to the correct diagnosis and it has been noted that cyst fluid of functional cyst is saffron yellow and these patients can be treated in a single setting where aspiration, fluid should be sent for cytological examination and also estradiol and progesterone levels. A high estradiol level (> 500 pg/mL) is suggestive of a functional cyst. Once diagnosis is confirmed a follow-up ultrasound is done after 3 months, and early if there are recurrence of symptoms.

If the aspirated fluid is clear, chocolate, dermoid or turbid, a functional cyst is excluded and an immediate laparoscopic treatment is necessary and surgical treatment is indicated.

PUNCTURE OF MALIGNANT TUMORS

When proposing a ultrasound guided puncture of adnexal masses, risk of spillage is always there and is also with laparoscopic puncture of these masses. The prognostic consequences are related to the delay between the puncture and delay in definitive surgical treatment. Studies have shown, that, if the tumor is not removed immediately, the prognosis of malignant ovarian tumor is worsened by punctural biopsy.

CONCLUSION

- USG guided puncture is one of the tool available in management of adnexal masses (Fig. 14.1)

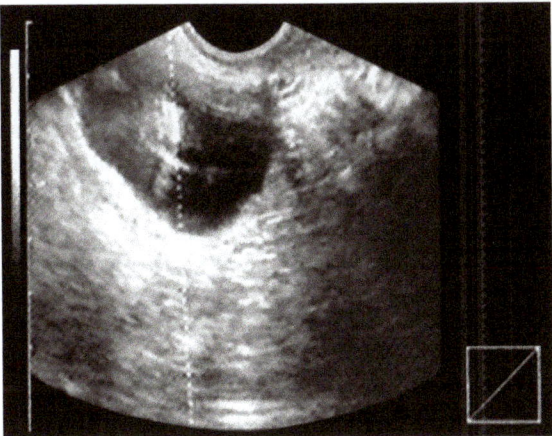

Fig. 14.1: Cyst puncture under ultrasound guidance.

- It should be used following strict guideline to avoid the spillage of unexpected malignant masses and benign ovarian should be removed surgically
- It is unnecessary for masses less than 2 cm (even in post menopausal women)
- It is possible if the cyst is functional (hyperstimulation, less than 5 years after menopause); if patient has undergone multiple pelvic surgeries and expecting extensive pelvic adhesions, mass is entirely cystic or with thin septae, if CA 125 is below 35, mass cystic and woman post menopausal
- It is not possible if cyst is not functional, patient has no previous surgeries or pelvic adhesions, mass is solid/mixed/septated or CA125 is above 35 and patient is postmenopausal
- USG guided puncture is sufficient if the cyst fluid is saffron yellow, E2 level is high and cytological examination confirms a functional cyst

- It is not sufficient if fluid is clear, dermoid, mucous or chocolate, E2 level and cytological examination exclude the diagnoses of functional cyst or if a recurrence is found.

The best indications of USG guided puncture are to treat:
- Functional cysts in patients who wish to avoid 3 months of treatment with OCP and/or follow-up
- Patients with extensive adhesions who either have a functional cyst or peritoneal cyst, already diagnosed or treated surgically.

CHAPTER 15

Transvaginal Sonographic Puncture Procedures for Management of Ectopic Pregnancies

Nonsurgical management of ectopic pregnancies include systemic administration of methotrexate, mifepristone or local injection of methotrexate, potassium chloride or prostaglandins under laparoscopic or ultrasound guidance.

The main rationale of performing transvaginal punctures are:
- Saves the patient from a more complicated surgical procedure (usually done under GA)
- Renders treatment as good as conventional surgery.

Advantages of performing transvaginal punctures are:
- The needle is placed in an accurate fashion within the target organ
- There is almost no injury to the neighboring organs as it is under sonographic guidance
- Technical skills to perform the puncture procedures are easy to master
- The ultrasound equipment is portable and therefore the diagnostic test and treatment can be offered in a variety of settings
- It has a relatively low cost per procedure
- The risks to the patient from the procedure are itself minimal.

When one engages in transvaginally directed puncture one should be familiar with two terms "slice thickness" and "free hand" approach for transvaginal punctures we need special automated spring loaded puncture devices that is mated to the vaginal probe.

PUNCTURE PROCEDURES

Culdocentesis

Before advent of sonography culdocentesis was the "gold standard" test for diagnosis of ruptured ectopic pregnancy. TAB increased the detection rate of ectopic pregnancy; but TVS with its high sensitivity to unique fluid in the cul-de-sac has significantly reduced the indications to perform a diagnostic culdocentesis. It is now indicated mostly to drain pelvic fluid collections such as peritoneal inclusion cysts and inflammatory processes resulting in abscess formation.

Technique

Culdocentesis classically was a blind procedure before advent of TVS.

The patient is placed in lithotomy position in reverse Trendelenburg position. Vagina is cleaned with betadine solution. The needle is introduced with TVS probe under real time sonography and fluid pocket is precisely targeted, without injecting air, all the fluid is aspirated.

TREATMENT OF ECTOPIC PREGNANCIES

The classic approach to ectopic pregnancies has always been surgical; the diseased tube, ovary or cornua end were resected and in case of cervical pregnancy; hysterectomy was the rule.

ECTOPIC PREGNANCY MANAGEMENT

There is today a non-surgical method for treating ectopic pregnancies which have not ruptured and where patients are hemodynamically stable.

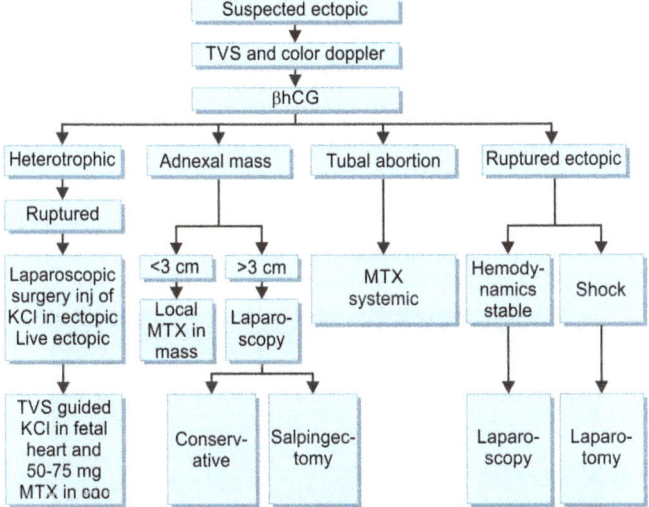

Technique

- Diagnosis
- Counseling
- Written consent
- Anesthesia
- TVS guided needle 17–20 gauge put in sac
- Salpingocentesis

- Injection of 50–75 mg of MTX or RU486 or others
- Prophylactic antibiotic
- Baseline blood tests and β-hCG levels
- Monitoring treatment by serial TVS color Doppler and β-hCG
- > 80% success
- > 70% spontaneous tube recanalization
- A very good, safe and effective treatment for early unruptured ectopic pregnancy.

SALPINGOCENTESIS (FIGS 15.1 AND 15.2)

Diagnosis of tubal ectopic pregnancy is made when patient presents with a positive β-hCG and on TVS an empty uterus with a typical adnexal "ring" or "bagel" sign.

The pre-requisite for transvaginal guided puncture and directed injection of methotrexate are:

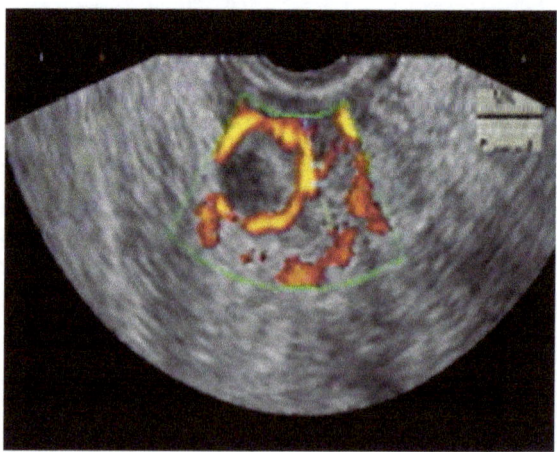

Fig. 15.1: Ectopic pregnancy as evaluated by a TVS and color Doppler.

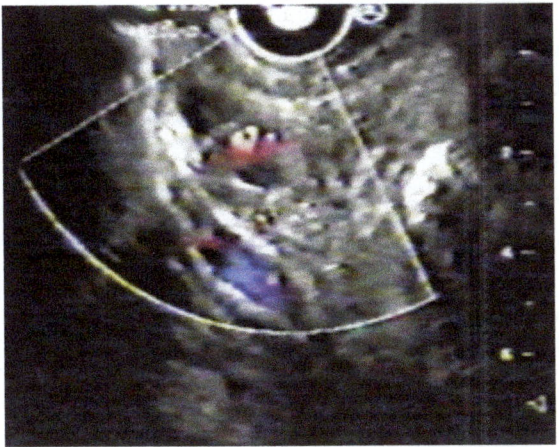

Fig. 15.2: Local injection in an ectopic pregnancy.

- Ectopic gestational sac must contain a viable fetus
- Menstrual age is less than 8.5 weeks gestation
- Tubal diameter ring should not exceed 2.5–3 cm.

The most important signs and symptoms of postpuncture convalescent period are:

- A relatively slow decrease of serum β-hCG levels when Potassium Chloride is injected it takes 30–80 days for the β-hCG to become negative and 10–35 days if methotrexate is used
- *Lower abdominal pain*: Between 3–7 days after puncture patient experiences lower abdominal pain due to uterine contractions as the decidual cast is expelled from the uterus or tubal abortion with varying degree of intra-abdominal bleeding if patient's vitals are stable and amount of free fluid in pelvis is not significant, patient may be followed up conservatively

- Transvaginal sonographic and color Doppler findings. These include an increasing distension of the hematosalpinx, increasing color vascularity and venous spaces.

Techniques

- Proper counseling of the patient is done regarding the procedure, risks and complications and nature of post procedure follow-up
- Written informed consent is signed
- Puncture is performed employing a 7.5 MHZ transvaginal probe covered with a sterile plastic sheath with a 21 gauge needle guide mated with it
- Patient is asked to void and is placed in lithotomy position. The perineum is cleaned with betadine lotion. A speculum is placed and vagina and cervix are thoroughly cleaned with betadine. Sterile drapes are put and sterile gel is used for good sonic contact
- A software generated fixed line is displayed on the monitor by which the exact depth of the ectopic pregnancy is located. If APD is employed, the depth of needle penetration is controlled by a centimeter scale located on the shaft of APD
- The patient is asked to stop breathing to prevent movement during inspiration/expiration and the needle is released. If a standard guide is used the needle is inserted rapidly otherwise the ectopic pregnancy will be pushed away from the field
- Before insertion of the needle, location of uterine artery and vessels of adnexa must be carefully established and care taken not to puncture them

- The target area is located near the fetal heart and methotrexate/Potassium chloride is injected once the needle is in place to stop cardiac activity
- As the needle is withdrawn, methotrexate is also injected into the placental bed
- Care must be taken, not to distend the already compromised tubes
- It is important to observe the pelvic structures and cul-de-sac following withdrawal of the needle and 2-3 hours after, that, for any complications especially enlarging hematomas.

CORNUAL/INTERSTITIAL ECTOPIC PREGNANCIES

Two to four percent of all tubal ectopic pregnancies are located in the corneal interstitium. Rupture of a cornual pregnancy causes a lot of hemorrhage and carries significant maternal morbidity and mortality (up to 2.5%). Treatment of choice is cornual resection which is only feasible in 50% of cases and in another 50% hysterectomy is unavoidable.

Diagnosis of Cornual Pregnancy by TVS is Done

- Patient with positive β-hCG
- Empty uterine cavity
- Eccentrically/laterally placed chorionic sac seen separately; more than 1 cm from the most lateral edge of uterine cavity
- Thin myometrium covering the gestational sac and also present between sac and uterine cavity
- No gestational sac visible above the level of internal os in longitudinal plane of uterus

- Presence of an echogenic interstitial line extending directly to the center of interstitial gestational sac (Not to be confused with bicornuate uterus)
- Pregnancy must be viable with a gestational age of less than 12 weeks
- Now viable cornual pregnancies with stable or declining β-hCG levels can be followed by TVS, with/without parenteral methotrexate treatment and β-hCG levels
- Satisfactory reports have shown that interstitial pregnancies are punctured transvaginally, contents aspirated and injected with Methotrexate and Leucovorin
- The β-hCG returns to prepregnant level in around 12 weeks
- The interstitial lesion has a rich vascular supply which persists for a prolonged period of time
- A trick to puncture the interstitial sac is to use a medial approach rather than lateral approach. Medially, the needle traverses the thicker myometrium and so at extraction, the needle prevents rupture or bleeding.

CERVICAL ECTOPIC PREGNANCY

Its occurrence is rare, under-reporting and lastly difficult to differentiate between a true cervical ectopic pregnancy or possibility of a non-viable intrauterine pregnancy in the process of passing through the cervix.

The new sonographic diagnostic criteria for cervical pregnancy:
- The placenta and the entire chorion i.e. sac containing live fetus must be blow the internal os (is at level of insertion of uterine arteries)
- The uterine cavity should be empty
- The cervical canal is barrel-shaped and significantly dilated.

The technique of puncture of cervical pregnancy is similar to that of tubal ectopic. The most feared complication is excessive bleeding, either at time of puncture or afterwards. It has been reported that a slow continuous discharge may be observed over the first 2 weeks of procedure.

CONCLUSION

Transvaginal route is a simple and accurate way to diagnose and treat different types of ectopic pregnancy.

The TVS puncture procedures avoid complicated surgeries, have low procedure complication rate, technical simplicity and ease with which it can be done as an outdoor procedure, have made these procedures popular.

It is also important to follow up the ectopic pregnancy treatment (puncture and injection of methotrexate/KCl) with β-hCG titers. After an initial rise, they plateau and gradually decrease to return to non-pregnant level within 3–13 weeks.

CHAPTER 16

Ultrasound-guided Transcervical Metroplasty

INTRODUCTION

Sectioning of uterine septa may be performed hysteroscopically with low morbidity and good surgical outcome. Using this technique, in order to prevent uterine perforation during division of upper part of septum both ultrasonographic and laparoscopic monitoring is proposed.

We can also do a transcervical section of uterine septa under ultra sonographic control without the concomitant use of hysteroscopy or laparoscopy (Fig. 16.1).

OPERATIVE TECHNIQUE

- After proper patient selection and counseling the procedure is preferably performed under general anesthesia
- The urinary bladder is filled with 250 mL of sterile saline through a balloon catheter
- An assistant places the transducer of the real time scanner in longitudinal or transverse position according to the need of the surgeon
- The uterine fundus is checked and bicornuate uterus is ruled out
- The septum is measured in length and width

Ultrasound-guided Transcervical Metroplasty

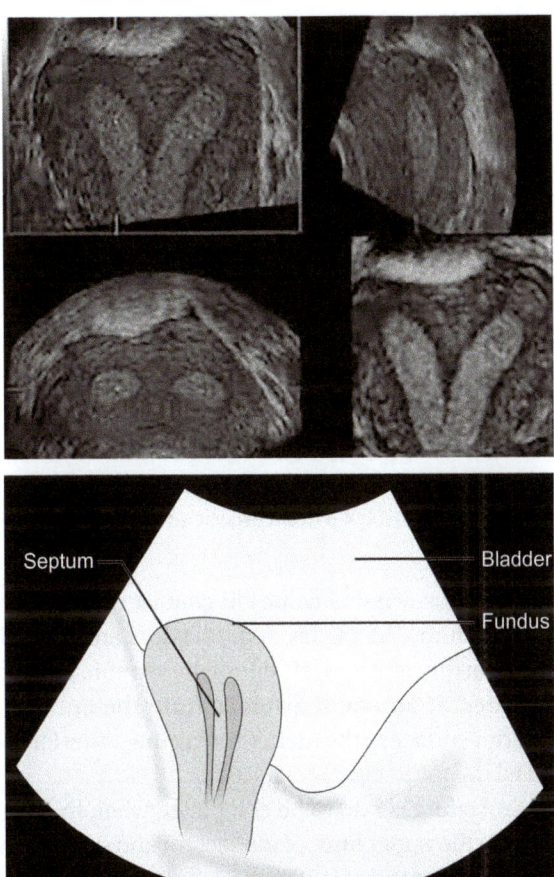

Fig. 16.1: Sonographic picture of a septate uterus.

- A pair of 4 mm diameter endoscopic scissors are used (Fig. 16.2). They are introduced into uterine cavity through the cervix without dilatation

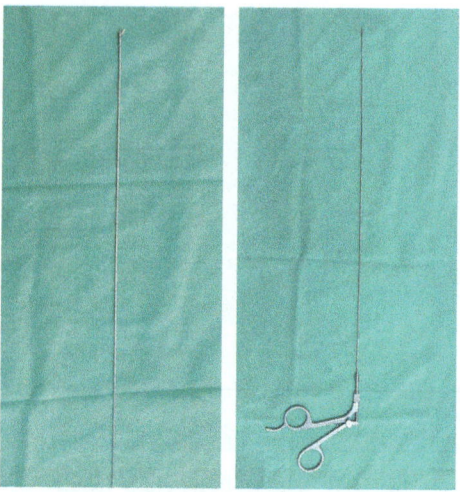

Fig. 16.2: 4 mm endoscopic scissors.

- The tip of the scissors comes in contact with lower edge of the septum. The blades of the scissors are opened and placed on the right and left side of the septum. The septum is divided at an equal distance from the anterior and posterior surface of the uterus, seeing the posterior serosal wall all the time (Figs. 16.3 to 16.6)
- The procedure is said to be completed when the distance between the upper limit of the section and serosal surface of the uterine fundus is 10 mm
- Usually this procedure taken 10 minutes and is usually a day care procedure
- Some workers advocate placement of an IUCD; a cyclical hormonal therapy for a period of 3 months is advocated
- A follow-up hysteroscopy is proposed following the withdrawal bleeding 3 months after the operation.

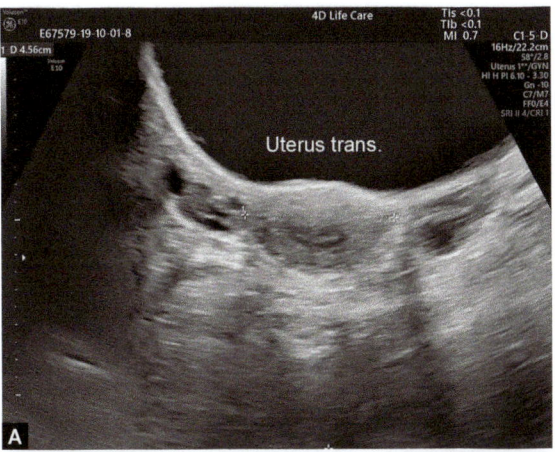
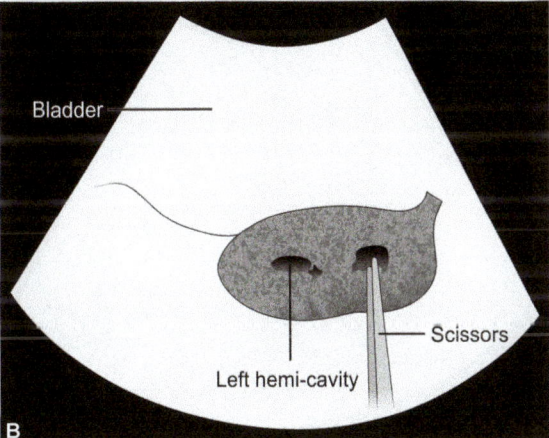

Figs. 16.3A and B: (A) Transverse ultrasound section; (B) Scissors are placed in the right hemi-cavity.

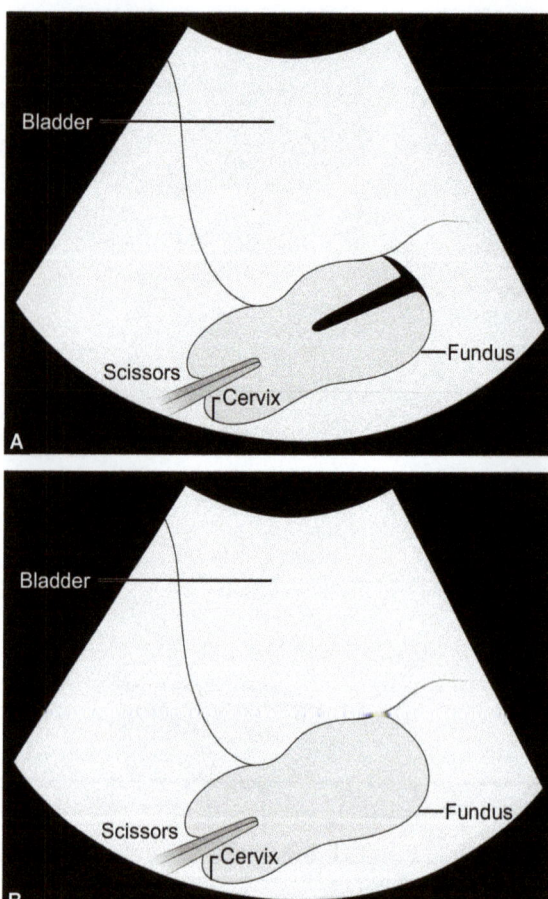

Figs. 16.4A and B: (A) Sagittal ultrasound section; (B) Scissors are placed at the lower end of the septum.

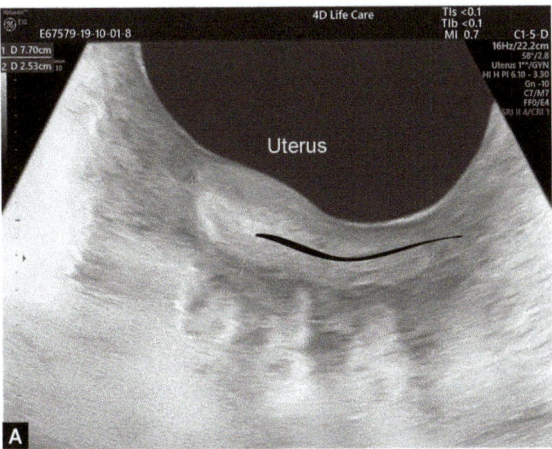
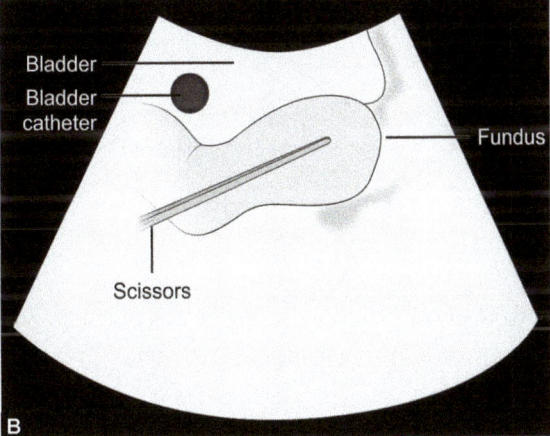

Figs. 16.5A and B: (A) Sagittal ultrasound section; (B) Scissors are placed at the uterine fundus, showing the thickness of the uterine wall.

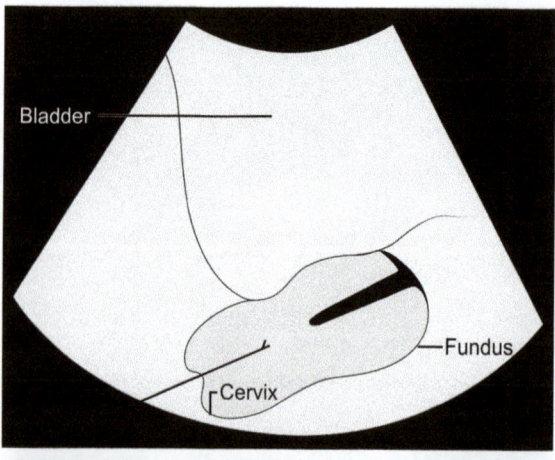
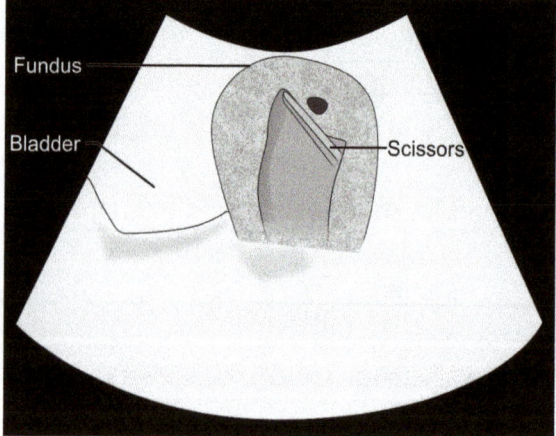

Fig. 16.6: Sonographic picture of opened scissors.

Postoperative Complications

- Bleeding
- Infection and discharge
- Arcuate uterus with residual septum
- Synechia
- Incompetent cervix.

CONCLUSION

Transcervical metroplasty is a treatment of choice for septate uterus especially in women with reproductive failure.

Ultrasound scanning enhances the efficacy and safety of the procedure as it allows precise checking of thickness of the myometrium left intact.

Secondly, as the procedure is performed without an additional laparoscopy or hysteroscopy reduces the morbidity and potential mortality.

Furthermore, it is a simple, safe, day care procedure with complications and risks comparable or even less than that with hysteroscopic resection.

17
CHAPTER

Infertility Procedures

Today transvaginal ultrasound is indispensable tool for the infertility specialist. Treating infertility without a transvaginal scan is like walking in the dark without a torch. A lot of infertility diagnosis and therapy is based on interventional ultrasound used in daily practice. These simple, reproducible, noninvasive methods help the infertility specialist to reach a diagnosis at the first sitting and counsel the patient. Interventional ultrasound has led to a one step infertility diagnosis protocol.

UTERINE CAVITY EVALUATION (FIGS 17.1A TO D AND 17.2)

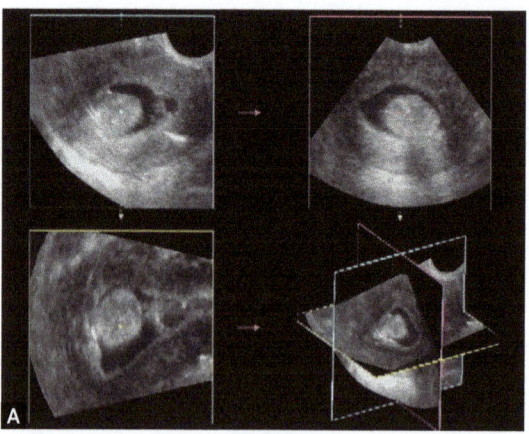

Fig. 17.1A

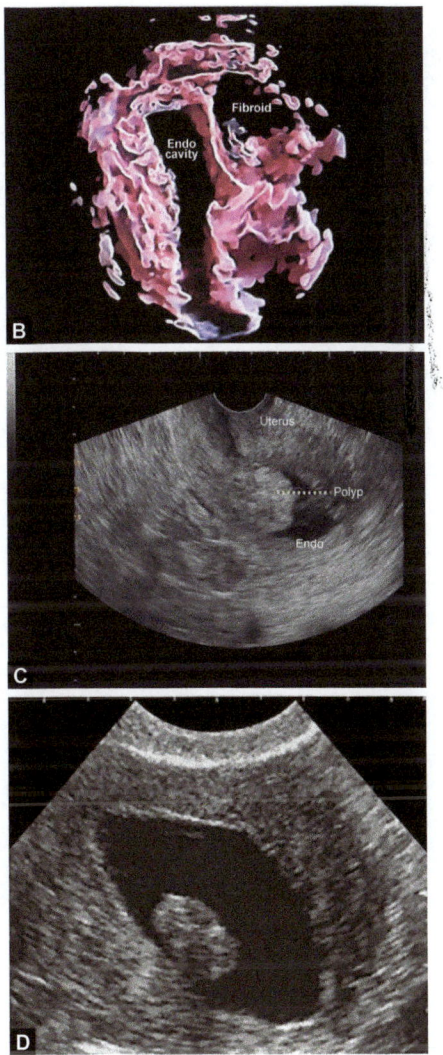

Figs. 17.1A to D: Cavity evaluation by saline sonohysterography (SIS).

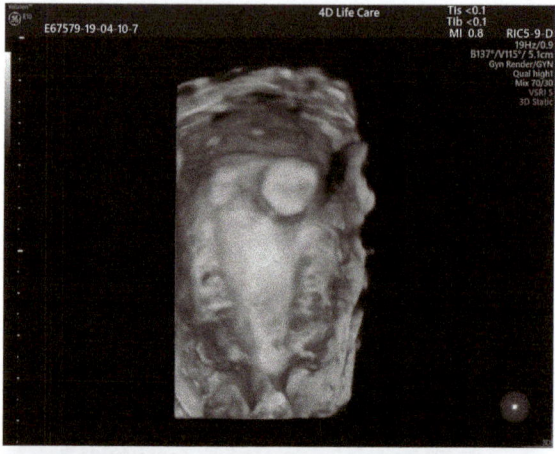
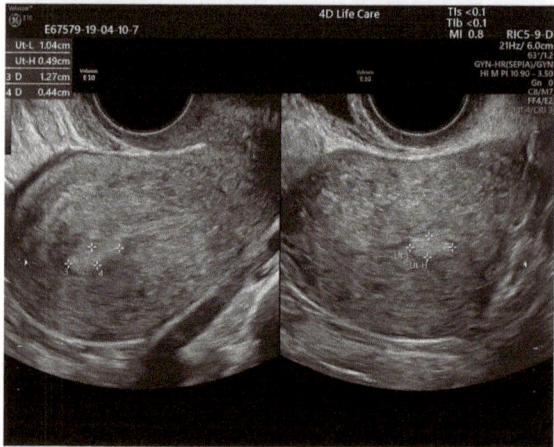

Fig. 17.2: Sonohysterography showing Asherman's syndrome and a polyp in the uterine cavity.

Infertility Procedures

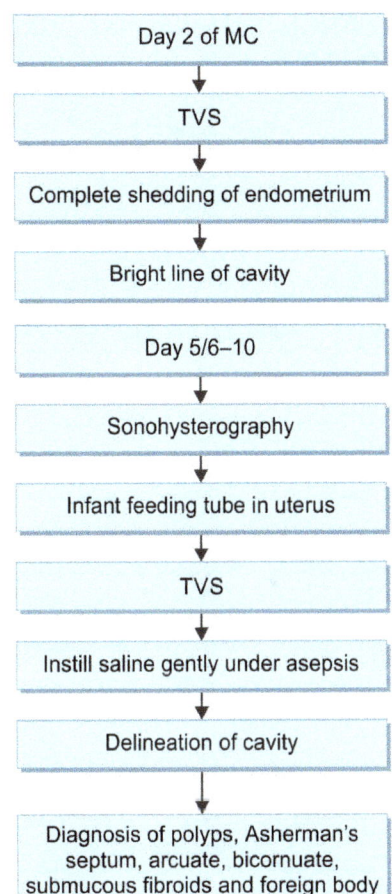

TUBAL EVALUATION (SONOSALPINGOGRAPHY) (FIGS. 17.3 TO 17.8)

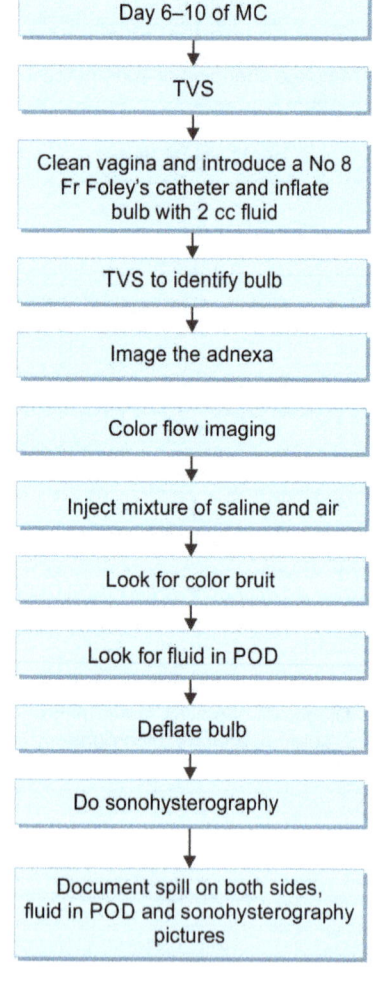

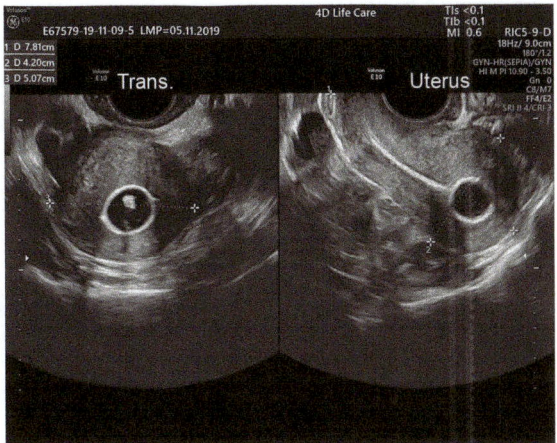

Fig. 17.3: Inflate Foley's bulb in uterus.

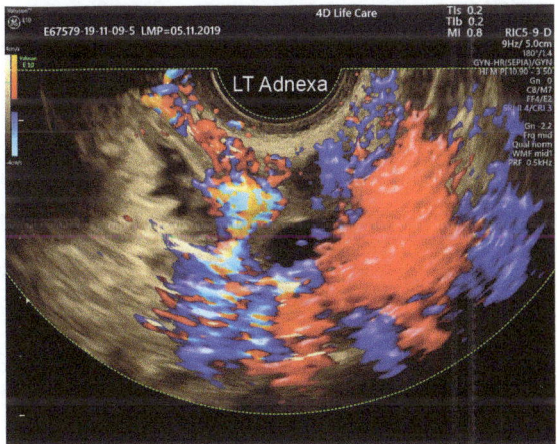

Fig. 17.4: Sonosalpingography color bruit indicating spill.

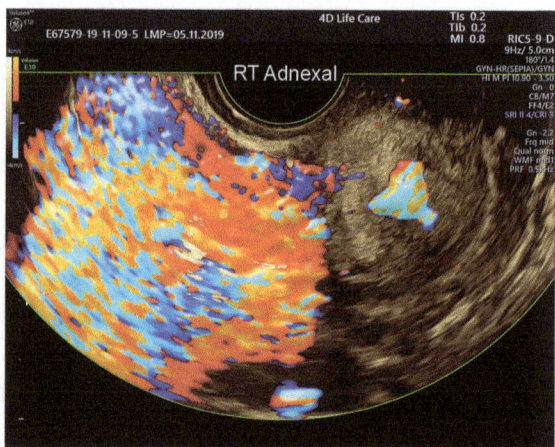

Fig. 17.5: Color flow bruit indicating patent tube.

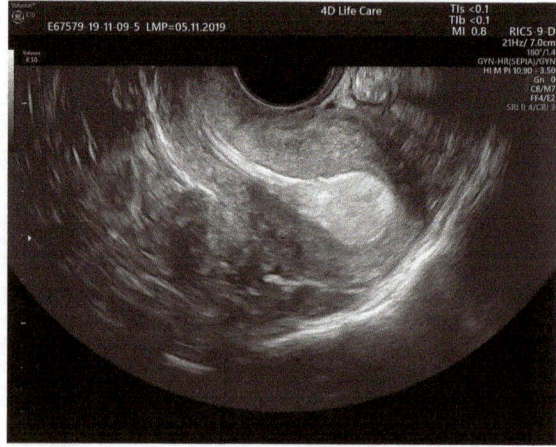

Fig. 17.6: Sonohysterosalpingography.

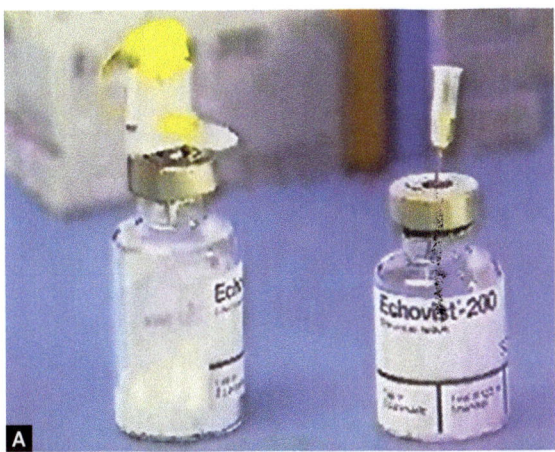
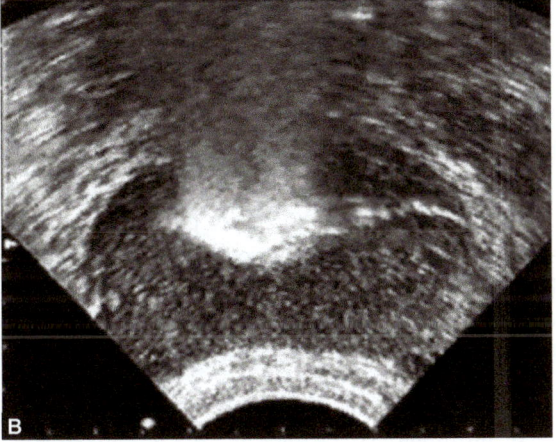

Figs. 17.7A and B: Positive contrast with Echovist.

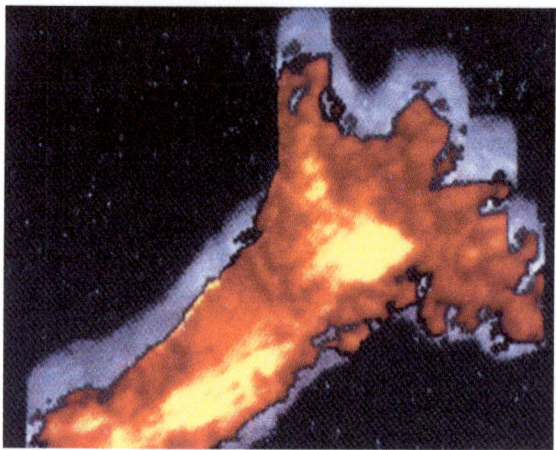

Fig. 17.8: 3D Power Doppler sonosalpingography.

OVARIAN CYST PUNCTURES

Ovarian cyst punctures: Many a times follicular cyst or CL cysts persist for many cycles and delay the ovulation induction protocols such cysts can be easily punctured under TVS guidance and the cyst wall sclerosed. (Technique described in Adnexal cyst aspiration).

OVUM PICK-UP OR OVUM RETRIEVAL (FIGS. 17.9 AND 17.10)

It is today unthinkable to retrieve oocytes by any other method than TVS guidance puncture for ART procedures.

Infertility Procedures

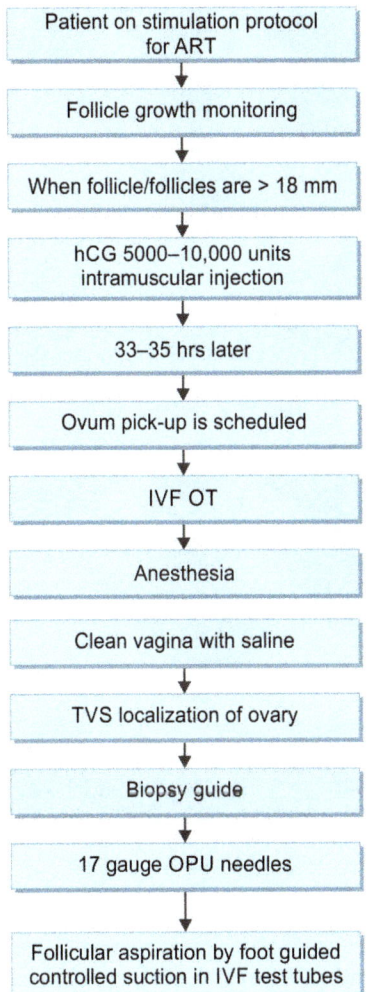

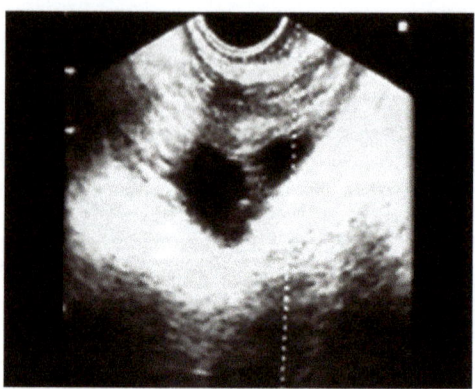

Fig. 17.9: Oocyte pick up.

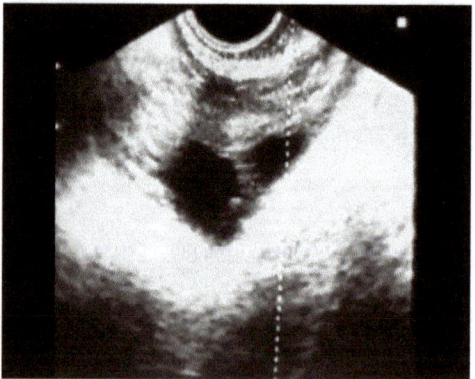

Fig. 17.10: Oocyte retrieval.

TUBAL CANNULATION (FIGS 17.11A TO C)

Tubal cannulation from the cornual end is best done by hysteroscopic guidance or fluoroscopic guidance. With ultrasound, using a Jansen Anderson cannula (JA Cannula), cornual cannulation can be done.

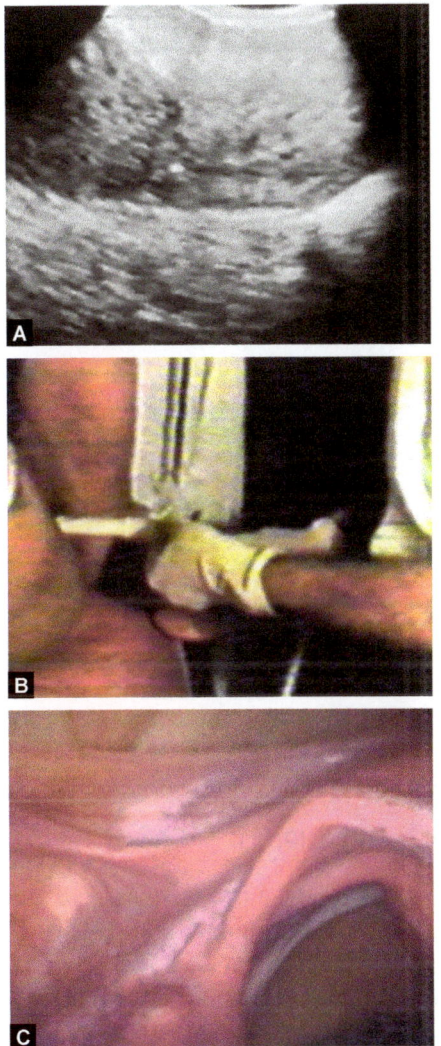

Figs 17.11A to C: Ultrasound-guided cannulation.

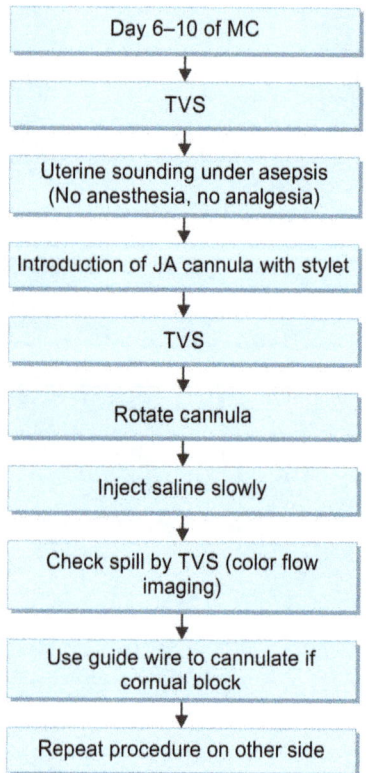

TVS GUIDED SIFT/DIPI/IOI

- Using the JA cannula a transcervical TVS guided semen intrafallopian tube insemination (SIFT) can be done in cases of single tubal patency
- Using a TVS guided puncture of pouch of Douglas a deep intraperitoneal insemination can also be attempted for repeated IUI failures with patent tubes (DIPI)

- Intraovarian insemination (IOI) into the dominant follicle 35 hours after hCG injection has also been tried as an insemination technique and is done by a 17 gauge needle through a biopsy guide attached on the TV probe.

USG GUIDED EMBRYO TRANSFER (FIGS. 17.12 AND 17.13)

In acutely displaced uteri and in difficult to negotiate cervical canal and internal os TAS is used at the time of embryo transfer to facilitate correct placements. A direct needle can also be introduced transmyometrial in cases when cervix is non-negotiable.

The needle is introduce from the fornix, into the uterus and the tip is advanced under TVS guidance to reach the endometrial cavity. The embryo transfer cannula loaded with embryos is then threaded in this needle and the embryos directly deposited in the endometrial cavity under vision.

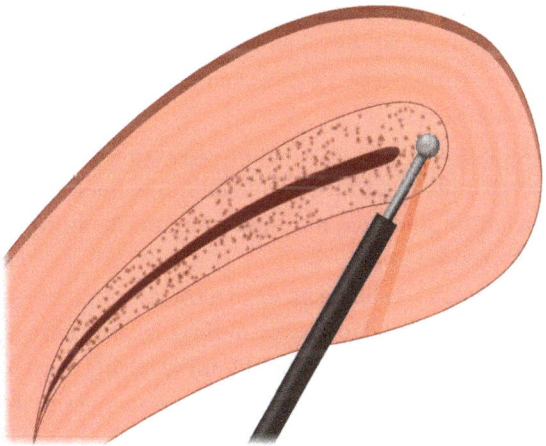

Fig. 17.12: Embryo transfer by the transmyometrial route.

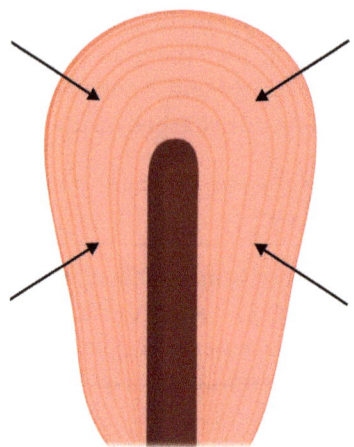

Fig. 17.13: Preferred routes to go via the myometrium in the uterine cavity (to avoid vascular injury).

USG GUIDED PCO PUNCTURE (17.14 TO 17.17)

Resistant polycystic ovaries, not responding to medical treatment are treated by LEOS (Laparoscopic electro ovarian surface cauterization).

Making multiple punctures on ovarian surface restores the endocrinology of PCO. The same has been attempted by ultrasound guidance multiple puncture technique after injection of some saline.

Also attempts are being made to retrieve immature oocytes from PCO patients and to mature these oocytes *in vitro* culture systems. This will save the patient from receiving injections of gonadotropins and will also save patient from potential OHSS risk.

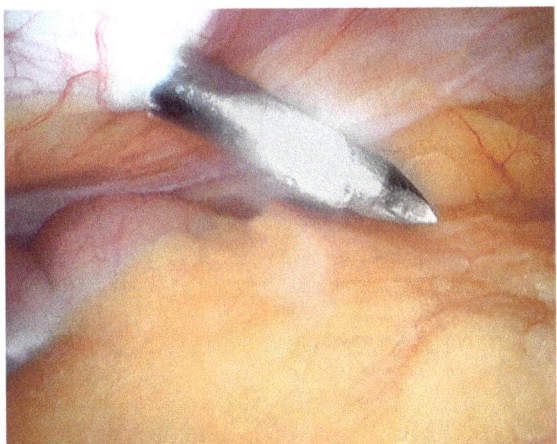

Fig. 17.14: Laparoscopic puncture.

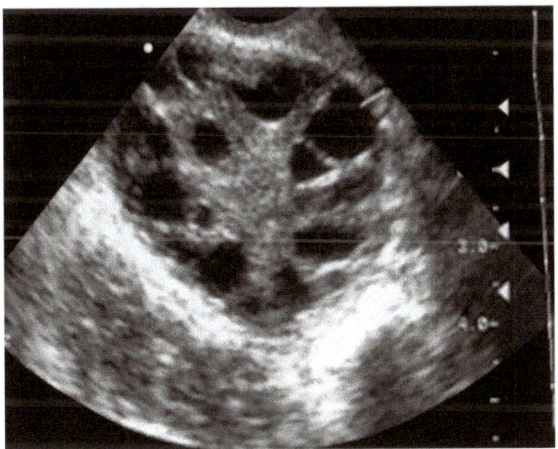

Fig. 17.15: PCO puncture by TVS guidance.

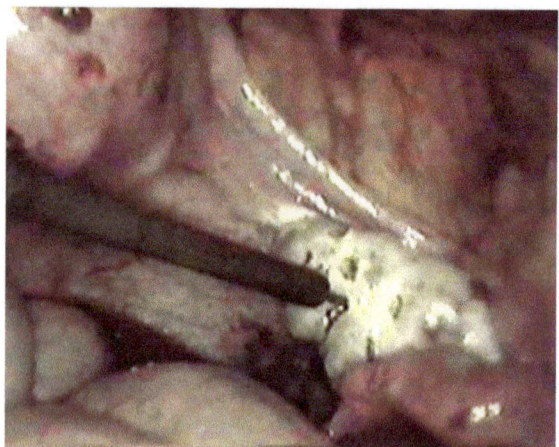

Fig. 17.16: Polycystic ovarian drilling by laparoscope.

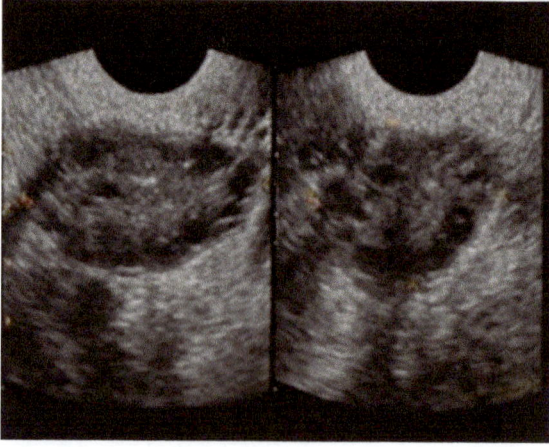

Fig. 17.17: TVS guided immature oocyte retrieval in PCO.

18
CHAPTER

Techniques for Assisted Reproduction

During the early years, in vitro fertilization (IVF) aspiration of the follicles was performed via laparoscopy, during the mid cycle. With the improvement in ultrasonic imaging, combined with the fact, that this method was less costly and does not require general anesthesia, ultrasound guided ovum pick up is the preferred technique.

OVULATION INDUCTION-OVARIAN STIMULATION

In an effort to increase the number of retrieved oocytes and to improve the success rate, most ART use some form of ovarian stimulation—clomiphene, hMG, hCG with/without GnRH agonists. Ovulation is induced by administration of hCG when one or more follicle is 16 mm and more in size, combined with E_2 levels of 150-200 pg/mL per large follicle. Follicular aspiration is scheduled 33 - 36 hours following hCG administration.

OVUM RECOVERY

Over the years different approaches to ultrasonic-guided ovum recovery has been suggested. These are:
- Trans - abdominal
- Trans - vaginal

- Trans – vesical
- Per- urethral

Transvaginal approach is the most widely used method.

TRANSABDOMINAL OVUM RECOVERY

One of the major disadvantages of this method is the use of general or epidural anesthesia as percutaneous ovum retrieval is painful.

An ultrasound transducer of a high resolution 3.5 MHz sector/convex scanner; 25 cm 16–18 gauge single channel needle which is disposable and a biopsy guide are used. A free hand technique is used for abdominal puncture.

Procedure

The ultrasound machine is covered with a sterile plastic sheet and transducer is placed in a sterile bag. The abdomen is prepared and draped.

The location and access ability of the ovaries can be changed by filling/emptying of the bladder and the puncture site is selected, infiltrated with 2% xylocard to the depth of abdominal wall.

The needle is inserted into the most superficial follicle in a brisk single motion and follicular fluid is aspirated using an aspiration pump with controlled suction of 100 mm Hg.

The follicle is flushed with the flushing medium and collected fluid inspected for presence of oocyte. Then the adjacent follicle is ruptured and procedure repeated till all the follicles are aspirated from the ovary and same procedure repeated on the other ovary.

Trans abdominal ovum retrieval is procedure of choice for ovaries adherent to the abdominal and pelvic side walls, but quite impossible if the ovaries are adherent to cul-de-sac/posterior wall of uterus.

PERIURETHRAL ASPIRATION

Patient lies in lithotomy position. The needle is placed in a side opening at the tip of a ND 14 Foley's catheter. The catheter with the needle are inserted into the bladder which is filled with saline.

The needle is advanced through the posterior wall of the bladder into the designated follicle and aspiration is performed.

This approach has been abandoned due to development of transvaginal approach which is easy, less discomfort to the patient and efficient method of oocyte retrieval.

TRANSVAGINAL OVUM RECOVERY

- Most popular method for oocyte retrieval
- Simple, easy and avoidance of deep general anesthesia
- Performed in operation theatre under strict asepsis
- Patient is in lithotomy position
- Need a good resolution ultrasound machine with a 5 MHz/7 MHz vaginal probe and a needle biopsy guide attachment and a suction pump. Disposable equipment includes—16 mL tubes of follicular fluid, catheter for embryo transfer, Teflon tubing system for follicular aspiration and a 16-gauge 25–30 cm long needles for follicular puncture
- Bladder is emptied by a catheter, a thorough cleansing of vagina and perineum is done with betadine lotion and then washed off with saline.
- The ultrasound machine control panel and transducer are covered with sterile plastic sheets. A small amount of

viscous gel is applied at the tip of the probe which is covered by a sterile condom.

- The aspiration set and needle are flushed with a small amount of flushing medium
- The probe is placed into the vagina firmly pressed against the fornix and the ovaries are visualized
- The target follicle is punctured by a swift movement, while the other hand keeps the probe firmly applied to the fornix.

As soon as the follicle has been entered the vacuum pump is activated and as the follicular fluid is aspirated, the follicle is seen collapsing.

- By proper manipulation of the needle, almost all the follicles are aspirated without taking out the needle
- Same procedure is repeated on the contralateral ovary
- Special precaution is to be applied to prevent puncture of large vessels (identified by rotating and observing it in longitudinal view) and an adherent bowel (identified by peristalsis)
- The tubes are immediately transferred to the laboratory
- The procedure is preferably done under a short general anesthesia. Paracervical block with 2% xylocard and vaginal puncture site with a sedative drug or epidural anesthesia can also be used.

Problems and Complications

- High positioned ovaries and distantly located fornices may make this procedure difficult. Placing the patient in Fowler position and applying external pressure on the abdomen, may make the ovaries visible and accessible
- Ovaries located behind the uterus may make the procedure difficult and it is best to avoid puncturing the uterus or cervix. The patient is placed in Fowler's position and ovaries

are swept with the probe away from the uterus and cervix in a desired position
- Bleeding in the cul-de-sac or the vaginal mucosal puncture sites is another complication. For this, after completion of the aspiration, it is best to aspirate the blood from the cul-de-sac and observe for a minute for refill. Vaginal mucosal site bleeding can be observed by per speculum examination such bleeding can be controlled by applying pressure or tight vaginal packing for few hours. Active bleeding may need a stitch, but rarely
- Reports of threatening peritonitis and pelvic abscess have been reported. These have to be surgically drained. It is best to use proper asepsis in the procedure and giving broad spectrum antibiotic 1 hour before the procedure.

TRANSCERVICAL EMBRYO TRANSFER

- It is a most popular technique nowadays
- The catheter is an open envelope and a tuberculin syringe are warmed in a CO_2 incubator at 37°C for about an hour prior to the procedure
- The patient is placed in lithotomy position after voiding
- A self-retaining speculum is put in the vagina and is cleaned with flushing medium
- A mock embryo transfer with an empty catheter is preferably done a day prior to the actual transfer
- Failure to pass the catheter is caused due to sharply anteverted or retroverted uterus or cervical stenosis. In case of acutely anteverted/retroverted uterus the catheter is bent according to uterine shape or hold the anterior lip of cervix with tenaculum and apply gentle pressure. Another option is to fill the urinary bladder with 500 mL sterile saline

- The selected embryos are put in a dish containing patient's serum
- The catheter is also flushed with the serum and then emptied
- The syringe is filled in the following order: 0.1–0.15 mL of air, serum, air bubble, embryos, air bubble and serum. The volumes must be kept to a minimum in order to prevent uterine contractions
- After touching the uterine fundus the tip of the catheter is withdrawn by approximately 1 cm and the embryos are injected
- After waiting for about 20 second, the catheter is withdrawn and taken to the laboratory for inspection. A small amount of medium is used to flush the catheter without bubbles
- The patient is kept on bed rest for several hours.

Alternative techniques are an ultrasound guided embryo transfer where an abdominal transducer is used to follow the catheter.

In cases of severe cervical stenosis, surgical ultrasound guided transfer is done when embryos are placed through a 16 gauge needle through the uterine wall under ultrasound guidance.

Secondly, embryos can also be passed through the cervix and uterine cavity and into the tubes through a flexible 5.5 French Teflon outer cannula with a metal obturator which is used to pass through the cervix and a 3.0 French inner cannula. The inner cannula is advanced into isthmic portion of tubes under ultrasonic guidance.

This approach allows access to fallopian tubes without need of laparoscopy and general anesthesia.

Appendices

Appendix 1: Ectopic Pregnancy Pretreatment Scores
Appendix 2: High Risk Pregnancy Evaluation Form
Appendix 3: Consent Form for IVF-ET

APPENDIX 1

Ectopic Pregnancy Pretreatment Scores

	Score		
Variable	1	2	3
Gestational age (days)	> 49	≤ 49	≤ 42
β-hCG (MIU/mL)	≤ 1000	≤ 5000	≤ 5000
Progesterone (ng/mL)	≤ 5	≤ 10	> 10
Abdominal pain	None	Induced	Spontaneous
Hydrosalpinx (cm)	≤ 1	≤ 3	≤ 3
Hemoperitoneum (cm)	≤ 10	≤ 100	≤ 100

For score 12 or less → Medical treatment 90% success.

PREOPERATIVE PREPARATIONS FOR INTERNATIONAL PROCEDURES

- All interventional USG guided needle procedures should be treated as minor gynecological operations
- Proper consent and patient counseling is a must for use of anesthesia and for the procedure itself
- Should be done by a trained sonologist (Gynecologist or a radiologist) who is well versed with the procedure and its limitations and complications
- Preoperative preparation includes tetanus toxoid injection, one dose of broad spectrum antibiotic (omnatax, supacef or magnamycin or augmentin)
- Proper disinfection of the part and site of puncture (vaginal or abdominal wall)

- Pre-and postoperative monitoring of vitals of the patient.
- Postoperative antibiotic cover is usually not needed.

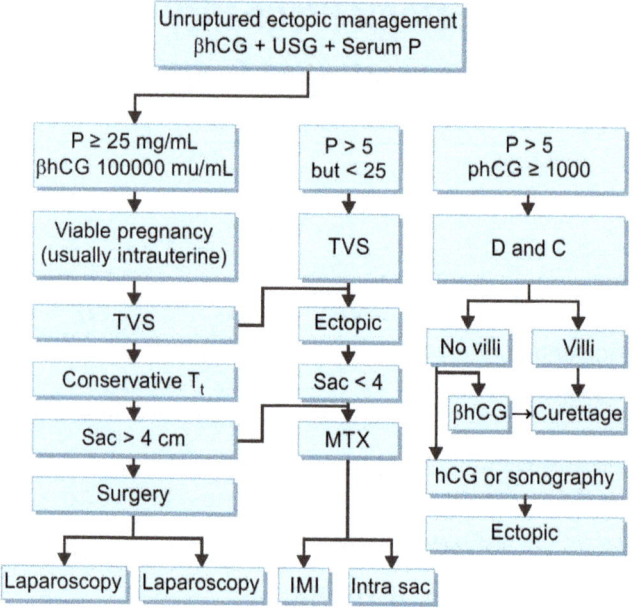

INDICATIONS FOR IVF AND OPU

- Blocked tubes.
- Failed repeated IUIs.
- Endometriosis.
- Oligoasthenospermia (Borderline male factor)
- Immunological infertility.
- Long standing unexplained infertility.
- Antisperm antibodies.

APPENDIX 2

High Risk Pregnancy Evaluation Form

Name ....

Age ....

Gravida ....

Para ....

Abortions ....

LMP ....

EDD ....

EDD by ultrasound ....

....

....

Prenatal Genetic Screening Algorithm

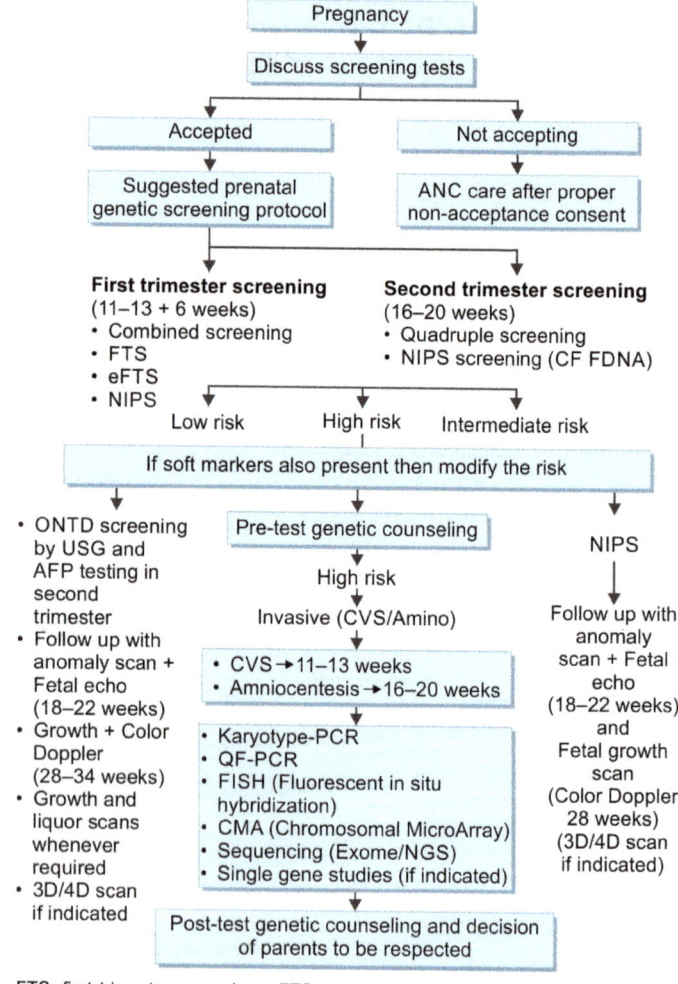

FTS: first trimester screening; eFTS: extended FTS; NIPS: noninvasive prenatal screening; CF-DNA: cell free DNA; ONTD: open neural tube defects; USG: ultrasonography; AFP: alpha-fetoprotein; CVS: chorion villus sampling.

High Risk Pregnancy Evaluation Form

Reproductive history		Medical or surgical associated conditions		Present pregnancy	
Age:	< 16 = 1	Previous gynecologic surgery	= 1	Bleeding	
	16–35 = 0	Chronic renal disease	= 1	<20 weeks	= 1
	> 35 = 2	Gestational diabetes (A)	= 1	<20 weeks	= 3
Parity:	0 = 1	Class B or greater diabetes	= 3	Anemia (<10 g%)	= 1
	1–4 = 0	Cardiac disease	= 3	Postmaturity	= 1
	>5 = 2	Other significant medical disorders (score 1 to 3 according to severity)		Hypertension	= 2
Two or more abortions or history of infertility	= 1			Premature rupture of membranes	= 2
Postpartum bleeding or manual removal	= 1			Polyhydramnios	= 2
Child > 9 lb	= 1			IUGR	= 3
Child <5 lb 8 oz	= 1			Multiple pregnancy	= 3
				Breech or malpresentation	= 3
Toxemia or hypertension	= 2			Rh isoimmunization	= 3
Previous cesarean section	= 2				
Abnormal or difficult labor	= 2				
Column Totals					
Total Score (Sum of the three columns)					

Genetic Screening Questionnaire

Name ....
Patient # .... Date ....

1. Will you be 35 years or older when the baby is due?
   Yes ....   No ....

2. Have you, the baby's father, or anyone in either of your families ever had any of the following disorders?
   - Down syndrome (mongolism)   Yes...... No......
   - Other chromosomal abnormality   Yes...... No......
   - Neural tube defect, i.e. spina bifida   Yes...... No......
     (meningomyelocele or open spine), anencephaly
   - Hemophilia   Yes...... No......
   - Muscular dystrophy   Yes...... No......
   - Cystic fibrosis   Yes...... No......

   If yes, indicate the relationship of the affected person to you or to the baby's father:

3. Do you or the baby's father have a birth defect?

   Yes...... No......

   If yes, who has the defect and what is it?

4. In any previous marriages, have you or the baby's father had a child, born dead or alive, with a birth defect not listed in question 2 above?   Yes...... No......
   If yes, what was the defect and who had it?

5. Do you or the baby's father have any close relatives with mental retardation?   Yes...... No......
   If yes, indicate the relationship of the affected person to you or to the baby's father: ....
   Indicate the cause, if known: ....

6. Do you, the baby's father, or a close relative in either of your families have a birth defect, any familial disorder, or a chromosomal abnormality not listed above?

   Yes...... No......

If yes, indicate the condition and the relationship of the affected person to you or to the baby's father:

....

7. In any previous marriages, have you or the baby's father had a stillborn child or three or more first-trimester spontaneous pregnancy losses? Yes...... No......

    Have either of you had a chromosomal study?

    Yes...... No......

    If yes, indicate who and the results: ....

8. If you or the baby's father are of Jewish ancestry, have either of you been screened for Tay-Sachs disease? Yes...... No......

    If yes, indicate who and the results ....

9. If you or the baby's father are black, have either of you been screened for sickle cell disease?

    Yes...... No......

    If yes, indicate who and the results:
    ....

10. If you or the baby's father are of Italian, Greek, or Mediterranean background, have either of you been tested for beta-thalassemia? Yes...... No......

    If yes, indicate who and the results:
    ....

11. If you or the baby's father are of Philippine or Southeast Asian, ancestry, have either of you been tested for beta-thalassemia?

    Yes...... No......

    If yes, indicate who and the results:
    ....

12. Excluding iron and vitamins, have you taken any medications or recreational drugs since being pregnant or since your last menstrual period? (include nonprescription drugs.)

    Yes...... No......

    If yes, give name of medication and time taken during pregnancy:
    ....

Consent for Amniocentesis for Diagnosis of Fetal Disorder

Amniocentesis is a test which can detect some birth defects and hereditary disorders. The test is done by withdrawing a sample of fluid from the bag of water surrounding the fetus (baby). This fluid is obtained by introducing a needle through the abdomen and uterus (womb). Some slight discomfort is experienced when the needle is introduced.

I, ..., have been informed of the following risks and limitations of amniocentesis for the diagnosis of fetal disorders, and have had the opportunity to question and discuss these with my physician and his or her assistants.

1. When the test is being performed in a stage of pregnancy when spontaneous miscarriage sometimes occurs, amniocentesis has not been shown to increase the chance of miscarriage.
2. The possibility of injuring the fetus or umbilical cord with the needle exists; however, the chance of this happening is considered to be very small.
3. As in all surgical procedures, there is a possibility of infection. If serious enough, this could cause loss of pregnancy. This risk is very low and every precaution is taken to maintain a sterile technique.
4. Ultrasound is performed to localize the placenta (afterbirth), and to visually guide the needle into the bag of water. It is also used to visualize fluid pockets and to evaluate fetal heart motion before and after the test.
5. In two-thirds of patients, the placenta is located on the front of the uterus. In these cases it may be necessary to pass the needle through the placenta in order to obtain amniotic fluid. This could result in fetal bleeding. Although fetal bleeding is rare, it has been known to occur.
6. It is rare that the test cannot be successfully completed because of an inability to get an adequate sample of fluid.

7. An occasional complication is leakage of either clear or blood-tinged fluid from the vagina shortly after the tap. This leakage is not considered to be a serious complication and it should cease within 24 hours. If leakage persists beyond 24 hours, it is recommended that you notify your physician.
8. In some cases, the fetal cells do not grow in culture after an amniocentesis and the procedure may have to be repeated. This occurs in not more than one in fifty patients.
9. Since the test screens only for selected birth defects, the results do not guarantee the birth of a normal child. It is understood that there is a slight possibility that the laboratory tests could incorrectly assess the baby's health.
10. I believe the benefits of my having amniocentesis outweigh these potential risks associated with the procedure. I have had the opportunity to discuss any and all questions about the procedure and give my consent to have the procedure performed.

APPENDIX 3

Consent Form for IVF-ET

We, ... (husband and wife), hereby authorize Dr .... and the team of the hospital and IVF center to treat us by in vitro fertilization and embryo transfer.

We understand that IVF-ET involves:

Administration of drugs/hormones for controlled ovarian hyperstimulation for obtaining adequate number of eggs.

Daily monitoring of egg development with blood tests and transvaginal ultrasonography.

Egg retrieval by a minor operative procedure performed either laparoscopically or under transvaginal ultrasound guidance.

Fertilization of the retrieved eggs in vitro, in an incubator, with the husband's/donor spermatozoa, transfer of the fertilized egg/embryo into the uterus.

Further blood tests and hormonal injections to support and monitor the outcome.

We also hereby give our consent and authorize Dr .... of the hospital and IVF center to perform the following operation or other procedure:

- Ultrasound guided vaginal oocyte retrieval.
- Diagnostic/operative laparoscopy and follicular puncture.
- Intrauterine embryo transfer.
- Laparoscopic intrafallopian gamete/embryo transfer.

We acknowledge that:

1. The nature and purpose of operation or other procedure and anesthesia, the risks involved, alternatives and the possibility of complications have been explained to us by Doctor ....
   ....

and all our questions, if any, have been answered to our satisfaction. We are aware that the practice of medicine and surgery is not an exact science, and we acknowledge that **no guarantee has been made as to the results that may be obtained**.

2. We further consent to the administration of such anesthetic as may be considered necessary or an advisable in the judgment of the medical staff of the hospital.

3. We consent to the admittance of observers, in accordance with ordinary practices of the hospital, to the use of Close-circuit television, the taking of photographs (including motion pictures), and the preparation of drawings and similar illustrative, graphic material, and we also consent to the use of such photographs and other material for scientific purposes, provided our identity is not revealed by the pictures or by the descriptive text accompanying them.

4. We understand that there is **neither guarantee of a successful outcome nor is there an assurance of a normal healthy live birth if pregnancy does occur**.

5. We understand that **failure may be due to a variety of factors** such as failure to respond to the ovulation inducing drugs, failed retrieval of eggs, inability of the husband to produce sperm, poor quality of eggs or sperm on the day of IVF, failed fertilization or a laboratory accident resulting in the loss of an egg or embryo.

It is, of course, understood that even after signing this consent form we may withdraw from the program without prejudicing our future therapy of clinical care.

Patient's signature .... Date : ....

Husband's signature .... Date : ....

I have explained the above to the subject on the date stated on this consent form.

Physician's signature ....

Date ....

Principal IVF Consent Form

We .... (the wife)
and ....
(the husband)..
of .... (address)
....

CONSENT TO TREATMENT FOR IN VITRO FERTILIZATION AND RELATED PROCEDURES

1. We have discussed the treatment and procedures with Dr ....
2. The treatment and procedures have been explained to our satisfaction and we have been given written information. We have been given the opportunity to ask questions which have been satisfactorily answered.
3. We understand that treatment may be provided by staff of the hospital.
4. We acknowledge that while the purpose of the treatment and procedures is to establish a viable pregnancy a guarantee of success cannot be and has not been given.
5. We acknowledge that the procedures may be cancelled prior to completion of a course of treatment.
6. We understand that there are risks associated with the procedures including but not limited to the risks of miscarriage, tubal pregnancy and multiple pregnancy.
7. We understand that fetal abnormalities may occur in association with the treatment and procedures as may also occur with natural conception.
8. We are aware that we are free to withdraw from the treatment programs at any stage.

9. If we have eggs which do not fertilize or are not inseminated, we request that: *(circle your choice)*
   a. They be made available for testing procedures not involving fertilization; or
   b. They be disposed off immediately.
10. If we have embryos which are not be transferred or cryopreserved because they are abnormal or of poor quality or surplus to our needs we request that:

    (circle your choice)
    a. They be observed until they cease development; or
    b. They be disposed off immediately.

Signed:

....
(Wife) (Husband)

....
(Witness: *(Witness:*
Medical Practitioner *Medical Practitioner or*
or Counselor) *Counselor)*

Date .... Date ....

Consent for Oocyte Donation

We .... (the wife)
and ....
(the husband) ....
of .... (address)
....

CONSENT TO THE DONATION OF OOCYTES, COH AND FOLLICLE PICK UP UNDER GA

We have discussed oocyte donation and stimulation and follicle pick up procedures with Dr ....

1. Procedures have been explained to our satisfaction. We have been given the opportunity to ask questions, which have been satisfactorily answered.
2. We understand that drugs will be used to stimulate our ovary to produce multiple follicles which will be aspirated under GA by USG guided needle.
3. We shall jointly determine the future management of any of our follicles.
   a. Donation of follicles to a couple selected by the hospital. If there is no suitable recipient, the follicles may be left to succumb and used for research.
   b. Disposal of the follicles. *(circle your choice)*
4. In the event that one partner becomes incapable of making and informed decision, it is our current wish that:

   (circle your choice)
   a. The other partner be given the opportunity to make lawful decision.
   b. The follicles be dealt with according to paragraph 4.
5. We hereby give consent for use of drugs to stimulate the ovaries for controlled ovarian hyperstimulation. We understand the small risk of hyperstimulation syndrome.

Consent Form for IVF-ET

6. We hereby give an informed consent for follicle aspiration under general anesthesia, we have been explained the procedures, risks and complications associated with anesthesia and the procedure itself.

Signed:

....
(Wife) (Husband)

....
(Witness: *(Witness:*
Medical Practitioner *Medical Practitioner or*
or Counselor) *Counselor)*

Date .... Date ....

Consent for Acceptance of Donor, Oocyte

We hereby give our free consent for acceptance of donor oocytes in case of failure to obtain oocytes from (wife's) Mrs .... ovaries. We have been explained about the procedure fully in my own language by Dr ....

....

We will bring the oocyte donor ourselves and would like to maintain privacy in this matter. All the responsibility of the donor legal or otherwise is our own. The doctor has nothing to do in this situation.

Sd. .... Sd. ....
Husband   Wife

Sd. ....
Witness Doctor or Counselor

Donor Semen

We hereby give our free consent for acceptance of donor semen from cryofreeze sperm bank. We would like to maintain privacy in this matter.

Sd. .... Sd. ....
Husband   Wife

Sd. ....
Witness Doctor or Counselor

Consent for Acceptance of Embryo Donation

We hereby give our free consent for acceptance of embryo donation. We have been explained by Dr. ....
....
about the procedure fully in our own language. We would like to maintain privacy in this matter. All the responsibility legal or otherwise is our own.

Sd. .... Sd. ....
Husband Wife

Sd. ....
Witness Doctor or Counselor

Admission—Discharge and Treatment Chart

No.:..........................
Name: ....
Age: ....Date of Admission: ....
Address: ....
Date of Discharge: ....

Diagnosis	

Case Proforma Sheet (Husband)

Name: ....

Age: .... Reg. No.: ....

Address: ....

....

Occupation: ....

Semen analysis:

Date	Lab	Count	Motility	Morphology	Other info.

Wash:

Andrological evaluation:

Treatment: Date: Date: Date:

Case Proforma Sheet (Wife)

Name: .... Age: .... Reg No. ....
Address ....
....
Married since: .... years
Present M/C: R/IR .... S/M/H .... PL/PF ....
Past M/C: R/IR .... S/M/H .... PL/PF ....
LMP: .... Dysmenorrhea ....
Galactorrhea .... Thyroid ....
Operations ....
Obstetric History: GPALE .... Details ....
Contraction:
IUCD .... OC .... Condom .... Natural ....
Years of use ....
Tuberculosis .... Asthma .... Diabetes ....
Hypertension .... Drug allergies: ....
Coital History: .... Height: .... Weight: ....
BMI.: .... Anemia: ....
Pulse .... BP: .... RS.: ....
CVS. .... Goiter: .... Galactorrhea: ....
Hirsutism: .... Cervix: .... Mucus: ....
Cervicitis: .... Day: .... Uterus: ....
AV/RV .... NS/>N/<N ....
S/F/M .... Fibroids .... TVS: ....
D_2FSH: .... D_2LH: .... PRL .... TSH: ....
DHEA-S: .... T .... E_2 .... P_4 ....
CMS: .... PCT: .... SCMCT: ....
Laparoscopy: .... Endobiopsy: ....
Histeroscopy: .... HSG: ....
ASA: ....
Previous ART: ....

IVF Proforma

Name of patient ....

Age: Wife .... Husband ....

Address ....
....

Phone (Res) .... (Off.) ....

History:
Infertility: Primary/Secondary
Duration: Years
Obst. History:
Menstrual History: LMP
Past history/Medical history
History of Surgery:
Past infertility treatment:
IUI: Times   Stimulation with
IVF: Cycles   at
Protocol used
Eggs recovered = Eggs fertilized = Transferred = Outcome

Examination:
   P: BP: RS/CVS: P/A: PS: P/V:

Investigation:
Male:
1. Semen analysis: No. of reports: Date:
   Count: Motility   Act.   Slugg.: Abnormal
2. Semen Culture:
3. HIV
4. HBsAg

Female:
1. Laparoscopy: date
2. HSG: date

Contd...

Contd...

3. Hysteroscopy: date
4. Sonography [base line] date
5. Hormones [base line]   FSH   LH   PRL   Prog.
6. EB: date
7. Hb   Bl Sugar   HIV   HBsAg   Urine

Suitability for IVF: Good: Fair: Poor:
Patient willingness: Good: Fair: Poor:

Anesthesia Record

Patient's Name: ....
Age: .... Date: ....
Operation: .... Diagnosis: ....
Preoperative: BP: .... Pulse: .... Hb: ....
                      CVS. ....
                      RS: ....
                      Others: ....
Premedication: ....
Anesthesia: Spinal: .... Needle No. ....
                      General: .... Intubation: .... Yes/No
                      Drugs used: .... Airway: .... Yes/No
                                  Pulse oximeter: ....Yes/No
                                  Cardiac monitor ....Yes/No

PREOPERATIVE OBSERVATIONS

Time	Pulse	BP	% O_2 Sat	Medications

Postoperative condition:
Pulse: .... Level of consciousness: ....
BP: .... General condition: ....
Anesthetist's Name: ....

Request for Registration

Kindly register our names at your clinic for consultation and advice of treatment for our infertility. We understand that treatment may involve any of the Assisted Reproductive Technologies such as Ovulation Induction with drugs and Timed Intercourse, Artificial Insemination, Intrauterine Insemination, in vitro Fertilization and Embryo Transfer, Zygote Intrafallopian Transfer.

Cryopreservation of Semen or Embryos, Oocyte Semen Donation and other forms of Medically Assisted Reproductive Technologies.

Name of Wife: .... Signature ....

Date of Birth: ....

Occupation: ....

Name of Husband: .... Signature ....

Date of Birth: ....

Occupation: ....

Address: ....

....

....

Telephone Nos. .... Contact No. ....

Referred by: .... Reg. No ....

Address and Telephone Nos. of the Referring Doctor:

....

IVF CHART

Patient Name: Date: / 202
Chart No.: Aspiration Time:
IVF/ICSI   PESA/ICSI   TESA/ICSI   Thawing ET
ED   OD   DS   Surrogate

Hormone Profile: Base line E_2:   PRL: P_4: β-hCG: LH: FSH: E_2 pattern:

Day of MC					
Date					
RO					
LO					
PIRO					
PILO					
RIRO					
RILO					

Hormones					
E2					
P4					
LH					

USSR					
Myom.					
Endom (MM)					
Zone BL. Vessel					
End. Peristalsis					
UTA PI					
UITA RI					
Score (UBP)					

Drugs for COH					

SPERM DATA

	Husband	Donor
Count (x10^6/mL)	( )	
Motility (Alive)%		
Activity Grade	I II III IV	I II III IV
Volume (mL)		

REMARKS

	Age	Wife/Hus.
Category		
Yr. of Inf.		
Cycle date		
Induction methods		

Consent Form for IVF-ET 189

Induction Methods

1. Combo
2. GnRH A (Short)
3. GnRH A (Long)
4. GnRH A Low Dose
5. Low Dose (CC/HMG)
6. Psure FSH
7. C.C.
8. HMG
9. Natural Cycle
10. Others (Anta)

Category

1. Tubal F.
2. Male F.
3. Endometriosis
4. Uterine F.
5. Cervical F.
6. Undiagnosed
7. Immunological F.
   - 1 : Male
   - 3 : Female
8. Anovulation
9. Others (   )

Embryo Freezing

Stage	Grade	No.

Date: /   200
Method

TRANSFER DATA

Date: /   200

Instrument	Rating	Complications	Catheter
Sound	Easy	Bleeding	Tom cat
Dilator	Moderate	Leakage	OCD
Tenaculum	Difficult	Pain	Wallace
None	Failure	Others	Other

EMBRYOLOGY DATA

#of Dish	No. of Eggs	Deg. of maturation	Time of Insemi.	Day 1	Treat IVFE	Day 2	Day 3	Embryo ZIFT	Transfer IVF

Septa and lateral metroplasty, hysteroscopic correction of 108
Septate uterus 137
　　sonographic picture of 131*f*
Shunt, types of 48, 49
Single needle insertion technique 74, 94
Sonohysterography 27, 140*f*
Sonohysterosalpingography 144*f*
Sonosalpingography 15, 142
　　3D power Doppler 146*f*
　　color bruit indicating spill 143*f*
　　color flow 28
Spina bifida 21, 23
Stress incontinence surgery and ultrasound 113
Surgery
　　abdominal 28
　　laparoscopic 28
Synechia 137

T

Terramycin 103
Thoracoamniotic shunting 64
Transabdominal chorionic villus sampling 72*f*
Transabdominal needle 71
Transabdominal ovum recovery 156
Transabdominal sampling 74
Transcervical catheter 71
Transcervical chorionic villus sampling 72*f*
Transcervical embryo transfer 159
Transcervical metroplasty 108, 137
Transcervical sampling 73
Transducers, selection of 79
Transvaginal ovum recovery 157
Transvaginal probe with biopsy guide and needle 98*f*, 99*f*

Transvaginal sonographic puncture procedures 121
Transverse ultrasound section 133*f*
Triplet pregnancy, ultrasound picture of 84*f*
Tubal cannulation 148
Tubal ectopic pregnancy, diagnosis of 124
Tubal evaluation 142
Tube 14
　　3D ultrasound evaluation of 101*f*
Twin pregnancies 93
Twin-reversed arterial perfusion
　　evaluation 46
　　sequence 97
　　syndrome 31
Twin-twin transfusion syndrome 46, 52, 95
Typical adnexal ring or bagel sign 124

U

Ultrasonography 6, 18, 26, 166
Ultrasound 53
　　physics of 31
Ultrasound-guided
　　cannulation 149*f*
　　embryo transfer 151
　　PCO puncture 152
　　prenatal diagnostic procedures 27
　　procedures, technique for 61*f*
　　puncture
　　　　contraindications of 116
　　　　indications of 116
　　transcervical metroplasty 130
Umbilical cord
　　catheterization of 44*f*
　　free loop of 42*f*, 43*f*, 46

Umbilical fetal abdomen
    attachment 46
Umbilical placental attachment 46
Urinary bladder study 112*f*, 113*f*
Urodochocentesis 64
Urogynecology 111
Uterine cavity 26, 152*f*
    evaluation 138
    polyp in 140*f*
Uterine movement 14
Uterine position 14
Uterine relaxation 57
Uterine septa
    sectioning of 130
    transcervical section of 130
Uterine shape 14
Uterine size 14
Uterine wall, thickness of 135*f*
Uterus 14
    arcuate 137
    congenital anomalies of 108
    inflate Foley's bulb in 143*f*

V

Vaginal probes 3*f*
Vanishing twin 89
Vascular injury 152*f*
Villi 37*f*
Viral infections 42

disorder, diagnosis of 170
immobility 57
injury 41, 81
invasive therapy 47
loss 41, 46, 81
lung maturity 40
medicine
    counseling in 17
    ultrasound-guided techniques in 59
muscle, biopsy of 32f
portal vein 46
reduction
    equipment for 51f
    procedure of 87f
    routes of 86f
research 25
respiratory complication 41
shunts 31, 47
skin
    biopsy of 32f
    instruments for biopsy of 33f
    needles for biopsy of 33f
thrombocytopenia 42, 46
Fetomaternal transfusion 41, 81
Fetus, medical treatment of 40
Fibroids 14, 27
First trimester screening 6, 18, 166f
Follicles, measurement of 14
Follicular development, monitoring of 15
Free-hand technique 39f, 40f, 59

G

Gastrointestinal tract 54
Genetic counseling 16, 69
Genetic screening questionnaire 168
Gestational age 163
Gestational sac 66f
    ectopic 125

Glomerular filteration 54
Glucose concentration 183
Ground glass appearance 104f
Gynecological complications 14
Gynecological ultrasound 14
Gynecology 12
    Doppler in 15
    procedures 98

H

Hemoperitoneum 163
High risk pregnancy evaluation form 165
Hydrocephalus puncture 48f
Hydrosalpinx 14, 163
    drainage of 101f
Hypercarbia 58
Hypercholesterolemia, familial 21
Hyperplasia, endometrial 14
Hyperstimulation syndrome, diagnosis of 15
Hyperventilation 57
Hypocarbia 57

I

Immunodeficiencies, correction of 46
In vitro fertilization
    indications for 164
    proforma 184
    treatment for 174
Incompetent cervix 137
Infection 41, 46, 75, 137
Inferior vena caval compression 54
Infertility 15
    and oncology 15
    immunological 164
    long standing unexplained 164
    procedures 138

Case proforma sheet
    husband 182
    wife 183
Cervical
    culture 69
    ectopic pregnancy 128
    polyp 75
Cervix 29
Chorion frondosum 69
Chorionic hematoma 69
Chorionic villus sampling 6, 18, 27, 31, 34, 50, 69, 70*f*, 75, 94, 166
Chorionicity, diagnosis of 93
Clomiphene 84
Coelocentesis 38, 38*f*, 39*f*, 65, 66, 67*f*
Coelomic aspiration 65
Coelomic fluid 65
Contraception, permanent 28
Contralateral lung, drainage of 64
Cord blood sampling 31, 42, 50
Cordocentesis 42, 45*f*, 64*f*
    routes for 44*f*
Cornual pregnancy 127
    diagnosis of 127
Corpus luteum, measurement of 14
Culdocentesis 122
Cyst 15
    aspirated material, cytological examination of 103
    pulmonary 47
    puncture under ultrasound guidance 102*f*, 119*f*
Cytogenetic diagnosis 40

D

Donor
    consent for acceptance of 178
    semen 179
Double needle technique 74
Down's syndrome 21, 23

E

Ectopic pregnancy 28, 107*f*, 108*f*, 124*f*
    interstitial 127
    laparoscopic management of 107*f*
    local injection in 108*f*, 125*f*
    management of 105, 107*f*, 121, 123
    nonsurgical management of 121
    pretreatment scores 163
    treatment of 122
Embryo
    donation, consent for acceptance of 180
    reduction 86
    transfer 151*f*
Endocoelomic cavity 65
Endometrial thickness, measurement of 14
Endometrioma 104*f*
Endometriosis 15, 164
Endometrium 14
Endoscopic cord ligation 97
ESGE classification 110*f*
Ethoxysclerol 103
Extraembryonic celom 70*f*

F

Fallopian tube 28
    abnormalities of 14
Fetal abdomen 46
Fetal
    anemia 46
    ascites 47
    biometry 13
    biopsy 31
    bladder aspiration 64
    blood
        sampling 27, 95
        transfusion 31

Index

Ovarian cyst 103f, 104f
    aspiration of 15
    injection of 15
    puncture 103f, 146
Ovarian stimulation 155
Ovary 14, 15
    abnormal 104f
Ovulation induction 85, 155
Ovum
    pick-up 4f, 146
    recovery 155
    retrieval 146

P

Pain
    abdominal 163
    lower abdominal 125
Parasitic infections 42
Pelvic abscesses, drainage of 15
Pelvic anatomy, normal 14
Pelvic masses 105
    differential diagnosis of 15
Perinatal fetal assessment 46
Peritoneal fluid, assessment of 14
Periurethral aspiration 157
Placenta 46
Placental anastomosis, laser
    coagulation of 96
Pleural effusion 47
Polycystic ovaries
    diagnosis of 15
    drilling 154f
Polyhydramnios 97
    drainage of 40
Polyp 14, 27, 140f
Postpartum uterine evaluation 27
Postpuncture convalescent period
    signs of 125
    symptoms of 125
Post-voiding residual volume 111
Pouch of Douglas 150

Pregnancy 96
    early 12
    loss 38, 75
        causes of 90
    multifetal 51f
    multiple 85, 86
    physiological changes of 53
Prenatal diagnosis 21, 24, 93
Prenatal genetic screening 166
Prenatal screening 18f, 19f
Preterm labor 75
Principal in vitro fertilization
    consent form 174
Progesterone 163
Puncture procedures 122

Q

Quadruplet pregnancy 52f

R

Real time ultrasonography 77
Red blood cell
    alloimmunization 42
Respiratory function 54
Rh isoimmunization 41
Ring of fire sign 107f
Rocket fetal catheter 49

S

Sagittal ultrasound section 134f, 135f
Saline
    infusion sonography 27
    sonohysterography 139f
Salpingocentesis 124
Sampling devices 71
Sampling techniques 73
Sclerosing agents, injection of 103
Selecting puncture site 78
Semen intrafallopian tube
    insemination 150

International Federation of Gynecologists and Obstetricians Committee Report 86
International procedures, preoperative preparations for 163
Interventional ultrasound 17, 26
　anesthesia for 53
　techniques, negligence in performance of 24
　tricks of 31
Intra-amniotic infection 40
Intra-amniotic injection, rapid diagnosis of 83
Intra-amniotic pressure 49
　assessment 50*f*
Intracavitory tissue 27
Intraovarian insemination 151
Intraperitoneal fetal blood transfusions 64
Intrauterine contraceptive device 26
　extraction of 15
Intrauterine exchange 47
Intrauterine fetal transfusion 46
Intrauterine pressure assessment 49
Invasive obstetric procedures 34
Invasive procedures 15, 31, 59
Isoimmunization 40, 81

J

Jansen Anderson cannula 148

L

Laparoscopic electro ovarian surface cauterization 152
Laparoscopic ovarian cystectomy 104*f*
Laparoscopic puncture 153*f*

M

Macaca fasicularis 41
Malignant tumors, puncture of 118
Meconium staining 41
Metabolic defects 40
Methotrexate 28, 124, 129
Midtrimester amniocentesis technique 78
Minor uterine surgery 27
Minute alveolar ventilation 54
Multifetal reduction 84
Multiple gestation 22
　amniocentesis in 81
Myometrium 152*f*

N

Narcotics 57
　intraoperative 57
Needle, placement of 39*f*, 43*f*
Neisseria gonorrhoeae 69
Nitrous oxide 57
Nonimmune hydrops evaluation 42
Noninvasive prenatal screening 6, 18, 166*f*

O

Obstetric procedures 30
Obstructive uropathy 47
Oligoasthenospermia 164
Oocyte
　consent for acceptance of 178
　donation 176
　　consent for 176
　pick up 148*f*
　retrieval 15, 148*f*
Open neural tube defects 6, 18, 166
Operative technique 130
Ovarian carcinoma 15

Index

Page numbers followed by *f* refer to figure

A

Abortion 22, 25
Abruptio placentae 76
Acardiac twin 96
Adenomyosis 14
Admission-discharge and treatment chart 181
Adnexal cyst aspiration 146
Adnexal cystic masses 100
   treatment of 115
   ultrasound-guided puncture of 115
Alpha-fetoprotein 6, 18, 90, 166
Alzheimer's disease 21
Amniocentesis 8*f*, 27, 31, 38, 40, 50, 77, 78, 81, 93
   consent for 170
   early 41, 80
   freehand technique for 39*f*, 40*f*
Amniodrainage 95
Amniofiltration 81
Amniotic cavity 82
   amniocentesis for diagnosis of microbial invasion of 82
   microbial invasion of 83
Amniotic fluid 83
   aspiration 80
   culture 83
   gram stain 83
   leakage 41, 81
   loss 46
   microphage derived cytokines 83
   WBC count 83
Analgesia 8
Anesthesia 8, 34, 102
   general 56
   local 46, 56
   record 186
   regional 56
Anesthetic drugs 54
Anesthetic techniques 55
Antibiotic 103
Antisperm antibodies 164
Asherman's syndrome 140*f*
Aspiration pump 103
ASRM classification 109*f*
Assisted reproduction 28
   techniques for 155

B

Benign masses, puncture of 115
Benzodiazepine 57
Biopsy guide 4*f*
   and needle, abdominal probes with 3*f*
Bladder neck, descent of 111
Bleeding 38, 75, 137
Bloody taps 41, 81
Bolus transfusion 47

C

Cancer, endometrial 14
Cardiovascular system 53

EU GSPR Authorised Reprsentative
Logos Europe, 9 rue Nicolas Poussin
1700, La Rochelle, France
Phone: +33 (0) 6 67 93 73 78
E-mail: contact@logoseurope.eu

www.ingramcontent.com/pod-product-compliance
Ingram Content Group UK Ltd.
Pitfield, Milton Keynes, MK11 3LW, UK
UKHW021827140426
5217IPUK00016B/1237